WUSHU

The Basics of Chinese Exercises for the Whole Family

Chantal Dupont

Astrolog Publishing House

Contents

Introduction

In today's fast paced and technological oriented society family life is not what it used to be. Families today have to juggle their careers, friends, perpetual do lists, goals, school, community involvement, and getting enough sleep. For the parents, children's activities always seem to have priority, work takes up most of their energy, and housework is never done. Families are hooked on remote controls, fast foods, video games and the internet. As a result, an increasingly large number of people whether in North America, Europe, and other major countries in the world have slumped down on their couches and stopped moving--literally. And it's costing them their health. It is important to stay fit in this highly charged environment with healthy eating habits and a regular fitness schedule. One has to become creative to get around these barriers, and most of all you have to make physical activity a priority for yourself and your family. There are many physical activities offered to combat this lack of strength, energy, motivation, and hectic lifestyle: aerobics, running, swimming, walking, yoga, etc., but nothing seems to target the whole family.

The intent of this book is to introduce you to 'Wushu' a series of Chinese traditional exercises and activities which will add to your family time together and help to keep the whole family active.

Wushu is an ancient Chinese traditional sport which has become one of China's valuable cultural heritages. It has a long history rich in content. Wushu has been developed and enjoyed by Chinese people for thousands of years, because it is of great importance in conditions and community where nature adapts things and only the fittest survives. It is science and a good sport.

In the past, Wushu was developed for the sake of military prowess and physical well being. Wushu was seen as crucial to a soldier's survival in the time of hand to and combat. Today, military function has faded and it has been organized and systematized into a formal branch of study in the performance arts by the Chinese, while it's physical welfare and athletic functions have become a dominant aspect of Chinese lifestyle.

Today, Wushu is popular among the whole nation of China, practiced by men and women, young and old alike. Many people practice Wushu to pursue health, defence skills, mental discipline, entertainment and competition.

One of the great things about Wushu is that it doesn't need to be done alone. By exercising together, family members can keep one another motivated, and to have more fun.

History of Wushu

Literally translated, "wu" is military, "shu" is art. Wushu therefore means the art of fighting, or martial arts. Westerners are more familiar with the term Kung Fu which actually translates roughly into "skill," and was popularized by Bruce Lee and Shaolin Temple movies.

First systems of Wushu aroused even before the appearance of the Chinese state, but there was not Wushu in full volume - there existed only military preparation, "war craft". In the beginning it had a form of dancing-military exercises, but later it became a military subject taught to all warriors. At the end of II century all individual preparation of a warrior got the name 'Wuyi'. This term was kept during the following centuries and became a synonym to Wushu. Wuyi contained Juedi (wrestling), Shoubo (hand-to-hand combat), and methods of weapon combat. Sets imitated hand-to-hand combat, weapon combat, and defense from weapon attacking. Teaching was based on a set a of formal exercises - Taolu - which were executed as solo, or with partners.

Over the subsequent centuries the introduction of Firearms slowly eroded Wushu as a military tool. Its continued development moved almost entirely into the civilian field from a military system to a family system. Skills were passed on from father to son, and any disciples were considered part of the family.

During the later part of the Qing Dynasty (1644-1912 A.D), Wushu was outlawed for civilians, for fear of supporting a counterrevolution against the new Qing Dynasty. In 1912, the Qing Empire was overthrown and replaced by a democratic government named the Republic of China. The restriction on Wushu training for civilians was removed. It wasn't until the New China or the People's Republic of China, took control of the government in 1949 that Wushu was integrated as a daily practice for everyone.

After the Cultural Revolution the Chinese government saw the need to bring back its cultural heritage and reinstated Wushu as a National Sport and supported it through its universities. Today, Wushu is also a performing art. The performance of a superb Wushu participant can captivate and mesmerize an audience. Also, with the upcoming 2008 Summer Olympics in China Wushu will be recognized as an official sport.

Philosophy of Wushu

A set of any kind of Wushu exercises uses a dozen to several dozen strict rules of attack, defense and retreat. The principle movements are followed by supporting movements: Stationary poses alternate with action during a set of exercises. Many of the movements incorporate modification of the original self defense skill in order to enhance the aesthetic qualities and fitness benefits.

Wushu or Chinese martial art is a general term embracing various schools of stylized combat used for health and recreation. A traditional Chinese sport Wushu pays attention to both internal and external exercises, with fighting movements as it main content. It blends elements of performance and martial application. Wushu training emphasizes quickness, explosive power, and natural, relaxed movement. When practicing Wushu one must combine flexibility, strength, speed and focus in executing the body movements. Wushu training improves physical ability, health, and willpower; it gives an individual an excellent method of exercise, a personal art form, a competitive sport, and a basis for self-defense and sparring. Wushu can be practiced in the form of a number of routine workouts for all ages.

Chinese civilization and its perspective of life are heavily integrated with nature. Their philosophy stresses the importance and the belief in the "Unification of the heavens and humans", a harmonious relationship between the environment and human existence. Wushu is the essence of Chinese civilization and is a major component of the Chinese social, historical, cultural, scientific, military, medical, psychological, and educational developments. From this perspective of harmonious integration, Wushu is more than just a combat readiness training. It is also a life nourishing, mental, spiritual, and educational training.

Harmonious integration, on an individual level, is about the integration of the whole person. The importance of the physical postures and movements are highly integrated with the vitality of spirit. Wushu emphasizes "training the muscles/tendons, bones, and skin externally; training qi internally". Qi, in this case, refers to breathing; and the internal energy controlled, regulated, and developed by focused intention. With the proper integration of the mental and the physical, the whole body can fully express powerful martial movements. When one aspect reaches the target, all other aspects also reach the target. All styles of Wushu emphasize this harmonious integration. Each style, of course, has its own integrated expression.

Their training stresses righteousness, humility, loyalty, honesty, trustworthiness, integrity, modesty, kindness, and courteousness. Students are expected to be ethical before learning the martial components of Wushu. With proper martial ethics and with the spirit of benevolence as a guide, Wushu practitioners are working toward attaining harmonious social relationships. Wushu, we train the physical to aid the shapeless; cultivate the shapeless to care for the physical.

The Art of Wushu

Wushu includes numerous varieties and styles of exercises that can be completed with weapons or bare-handed, with or without a partner, and their great for all ages. Traditionally there are two schools –: Waijia the 'external' family (outer body workouts) and Neijia the 'internal' family (inner body workouts). The schools of Waijia concentrate on developing stamina, agility, physical force, strengthening of body parts exposed to strikes. The Neijia schools give priority to psycho-physical training and qigong (mastering of qi). Using a metaphor, Waijia is training of body and Neijia is training of spirit. Such a division is rather relative, because every school of Wushu has these two sides of training. The matter is the proportion between them. Traditionally, external schools are under influence of Buddhism; internal schools are inspired by Taoism. The external families are more vigorous and demand more stamina whereas the internal families emphasize graceful fluid movements.

Most Wushu arts are classified as external, and only very few as internal. It can be said (simplifying the issue a bit) that external styles concentrate more on typical physical training and typical use of force, while internal styles concentrate rather on working with co-ordination between mind and body and a kind of rather uncommon generating of power with use of whole, quite relaxed body. Some traditional theories talk about this as "using power of bones and tendons and not muscles". There is a lot of discussion regarding the difference between external/typical and internal use of force, as some representatives of styles generally classified as external claim that they are using similar kind of generating force.

The approach of Waijia external practice is to increase human natural ability. The basic human abilities for fighting are speed, force, and natural (normal) reaction. All skills follow these abilities. People want to increase absolute speed and force. Waijia skill training is designed and developed based on the body's natural reaction, what is often referred to as moving externally. From this standpoint it is relatively direct and clear for people to understand this way of training.

The approach of Neijia internal practice is to change the human natural ability. Neijia practitioners consider that changing the human natural ability is much more important than to increase it. Neijia people want to be quick and powerful in relative ways. They also want to change their natural reaction by training directed by the mind, what is often referred to as moving internally. Although there are some practices in Neijia for increasing the human ability too, compared to changing, increasing the natural ability is always secondary in importance and desirability. Thus there are many things that are not direct and clear, and even too difficult for people to understand.

Neijia and Waijia are two big branches of the Art of Wushu tree which offer us different ways to understand Wushu. One cannot say one is better than the other, but one can say which one is better for one's understanding. There is no better style but there are better practitioners. The most important thing is to find out which one is more suitable for you and your family depending on your personal characteristics and body condition.

Waijia Outer Body Workouts

The external forms of exercises are vigorous and forceful. The Chinese call these 'silk exercises or baduanjin' which means eight-section brocade. They are called silk exercises because for centuries working people have compared them to the qualities of silk brocade. They are a set of repetitive spiral movement exercises with emphasis on ground connection, waist connection, knee alignment, sinking, opening and closing of joints and rotation. These exercises will increase the mobility of body joints and relax the muscles and tendons of the practitioner. The spiral movements will open up and exercise the 18 major joints (in sequence from the head to the ankles) of the body, promote muscle relaxation and flexibility, and reduce physical tension and strain. One must concentrate on your muscles that they are firm yet supple, and this can be achieved by relaxing your muscles and nerves and then lightly tightening them when moving. Breathing should be natural and even throughout all these exercises.

The four systems of the basic workouts for the family are introduced here, divided into 35 exercises. The first 3 systems are divided are done standing and the last system sitting down.

The Four Systems of the Basic Workouts

System One

1. Pressing the Heavens with Two Hands

Stand with feet shoulder width apart and arms hanging loosely on your side. Breathe in, lift your arms up, as they come above the head turn the palms out so the fingers are facing inwards, with the back of the hands just above the crown of your head. As you breathe out straighten the arms, pushing up with the hands as if pushing against a ceiling, at the same time press your feet firmly to the ground. Repeat the whole cycle for a minute. This regulates the internal organs. It also relieves fatigue and increases inhalation's as well as invigorating the muscles and bones of your back and waist, it has also been found to help correct poor posture of the backhand shoulders. This exercise combined with drawing the bow to the left and to the right and shaking the body is beneficial to women who suffer from PMS including painful periods. The flow of Chi is enhanced allowing adjustment of hormonal and internal physical changes. Repeat this cycle 4 times.

2. Drawing the Bow

Step to left and bend your knees to assume a horse riding position. Bend the elbows and lift the arms up so the palms face your chest. Turn the left palm out to the left with fingers pointing up. Imagine the left arm is pushing against a wooden part of an archer's bow whilst the right fingers are curled around the bows string. As you breathe out pull the imaginary string to the right and push out with the left palm to the left. Breathe in and bring the palm back in front of the chest and then repeat the exercise to the right. This exercise is most beneficial to the thoracic cavity-the chest. It improves the circulation in the area. Hold the position for 2 minutes. Additionally it also enhances the flow of Chi in the small intestine. Repeat this cycle 4 times.

3. Holding up a Single Hand

Stand straight, feet shoulder apart, arms by your sides. Breathe in and raise your hands to chest level, palms facing you. Turn your left palm down with the fingers pointing backwards. Breathe out and push up with the right palm and down with the left straightening the elbows. Bring the arms back in front of you with the palms facing the chest and this time push up with the left and down with the right. This exercise increases the flow of chi on both sides of your body it benefits your liver, gall bladder, spleen and stomach. The movements of this exercise prevent diseases of the gastrointestinal tract. Repeat this cycle 4 times.

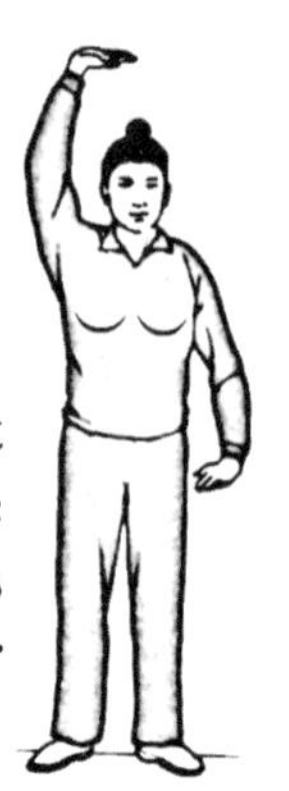

4. Looking Back like a Cow Gazing at the Moon

Stand to attention, palms lightly touching thighs. Lift the arms to chest level, palms facing you. As you breathe out turn the upper body to the left simultaneously turn the palms outwards as if pushing against a big balloon. When you have turned as far left as you can make sure the hands are still opposite the chest, hold the position for a second. Breathe out & lower the hands back to the Wu Chi position. Breathe in & bring the hands up and repeat the twist to the right. This is regarded as a very powerful exercise as it has a very strong effect on the central nervous system and the circulation of blood and Chi to the head. It inspires the power of the kidneys: Strengthens the activity of the eyeballs, neck and shoulder muscles. It also helps relieve high blood pressure and hardening of the arteries. Repeat this cycle 4 times.

5. Lowering the Head and the Hips

Standing in attention with your legs slightly apart and raise your right hand up in an arc above your head with the palm facing down. Breathe in and bend over to your left, letting your left arm hang loose to your left. Transfer all your body weight to the right leg, start breathing out and reach over the left to the furthest point that feels comfortable to you. Breathe in and straighten up with your right still in arch above your head. Breathe out as you lower your right arm. Breathe in and raise your left arm in an arch over your head and repeat the stretch. This exercise reduces tension in the sympathetic nervous system and effectively relaxes the whole body, enabling Chi to flow with ease. It also prevents fever. Repeat this cycle 4 times.

6. Touching the Toes with Both Hands

Standing to attention breathe in and raise both arms to the sides, palms facing up to shoulder level, then, up above your head. As you start to breathe out turn the palms face down and bring the arms down, outstretched in front of you at shoulder level. as the arm circle downwards in front of you, bend the knees as if going into a squat at half squat position, hold for a second. At this point each hand should be outside each knee. Start to breathe in and straighten up slowly, continuing to circle with your hand behind you, bringing them up over head and finishing with them outstretched in front of you at shoulder level. At this point you should be standing up, continue the cycle for a minute. This exercise stretches the spine and benefits the muscles of the lower back and legs. It is also beneficial to the internal organs of the lower abdomen. It strengthen the Kidneys, Adrenal Glands, the Arteries and veins. Repeat this cycle 4 times.

7. Clenching the Fist

Stand with legs wide apart bending the knees and form a fist with each hand, folding your thumbs inside your fists. The elbows should be bent such that the fist are facing upend resting on each side of your waist. Breathe out slowly as you extend your left arm in front of you at shoulder level, turning the fist over to finish face down. Start to breathe in and as you pull your right elbow back, extend the right arms you did with the left. Continue to alternately breathe and extend the arms in this way for **a minute.** Clenching the fist allows the flow of Chi through the entire body, right from the feet and to the hands and eyes. It stimulates the cerebral cortex and heightens the circulation **of** blood and oxygen in the cardiovascular syst**em.** Repeat this cycle 4 times.

8. Shaking the Body

Bend knees to assume a horse riding position with legs wide apart, place hands on thighs, thumbs pointing upwards. Next, breathe in and place the backs of your hands on your lower back, closing your bowels. Shake your whole body by bouncing up and down gently, breathing out on each bounce. This exercise allows the internal organs to massage each other. It is very good for the spine, the nervous system and sense of balance. When combined with Holding the Balloon and Looking Back like a Cow it is used to relieve headaches. Repeat this cycle 4 times.

System Two

9. Pressing the Heavens with Two Hands

Stand with feet shoulder width apart and arms hanging loosely on your side. Breathe in, lift your arms up, and as they come above the head turn the palms out so the fingers are facing inwards, with the back of the hands just above the crown of your head. As you breathe out straighten the arms, pushing up with the hands as if pushing against a ceiling, at the same time press your feet firmly to the ground. Keep arms straight, turn palms up and bend head back. Keeping eyes on back of hands; at the same time keep legs tightly together, lift heels, stretch body and breathe in. Turn palms over and relax arms; at the same time lower heels but do not touch ground and breathe out. Next relax and bring heels to the ground. Then breathe in and lower the arms by bending the elbows and bringing the back of your hands just above the crown. Repeat this cycle 4 times.

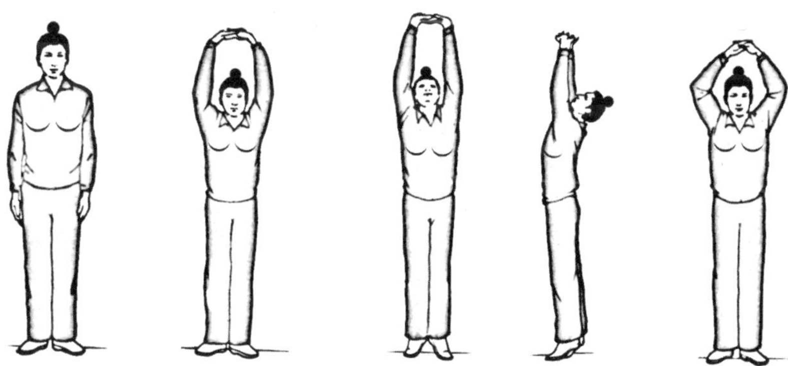

10. Drawing the Bow

Step to left and bend your knees and assume a horse riding position. Keep body straight and head up. Keep your upper body straight and thighs parallel to the ground. Bend arms into body at shoulder level, extend middles finger and forefinger into left hand, curl thumb and middle finger in right hand clench all other fingers. Imagine that you are holding the string of a bow, fingers on the string and above and below the arrow, and then pulling on the bow string with your right arm. Look to the left. As you draw the bow and string apart breathe in deeply. Aim the bow and arrow, and then release the fingers of the right hand to let the arrow fly. As you release the arrow, begin to slowly breathe out. Relax. Repeat this cycle 4 times.

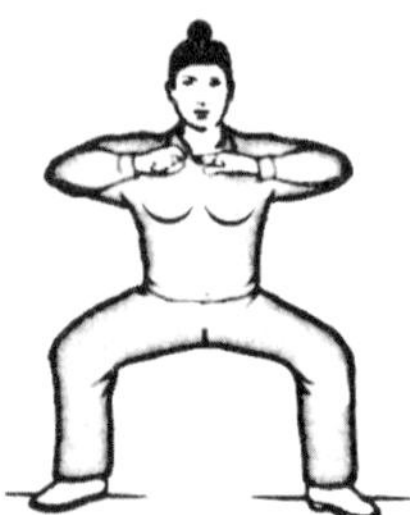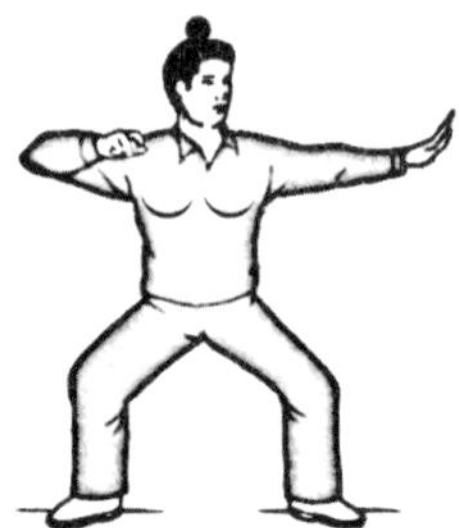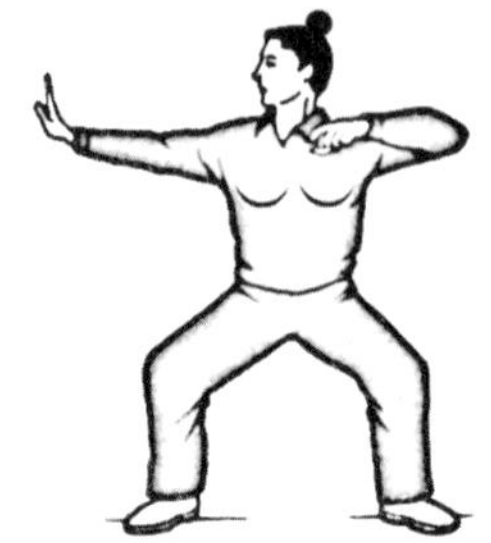

11. Holding up a Single Hand

Stand straight, feet shoulder apart, arms by your sides. Breathe in and raise your hands to chest level, palms facing you. Turn your left palm down with the fingers pointing backwards. Breathe out and push up with the right palm and down with the left straightening the elbows. Bring the arms back in front of you with the palms facing the chest and this time push up with the left and down with the right.

Raise the left hand above the head, palm up, fingers pointing to the right at the same time press right hand down, point fingers straight ahead and breathe in. Bend both arms until back of left hand touches top of head and right hand reaches rib cage and breathe out deeply. Repeat for by raising right hand and press left hand down. Repeat several times until you can speed it up and then repeat the cycle 4 times.

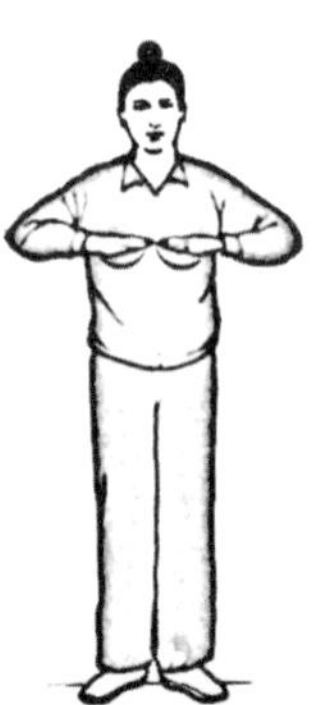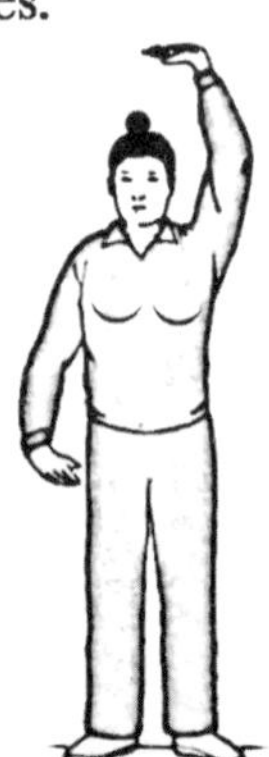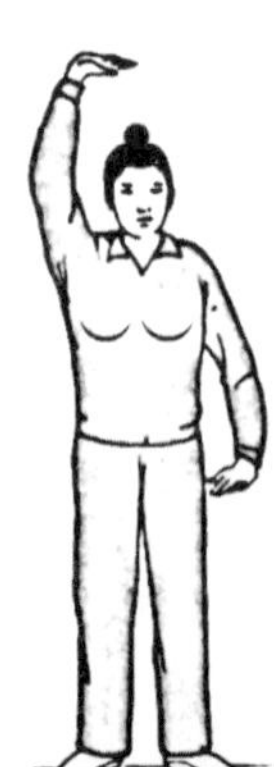

12. Looking back Like a Cow Gazing at the Moon

Stand to attention, palms lightly touching thighs. Lift the arms to chest level, palms facing you. As you breathe out turn the upper body to the left simultaneously turn the palms outwards as if pushing against a big balloon. When you have turned as far left as you can make sure the hands are still opposite the chest, hold the position for a second. Breathe out & lower the hands back to the thighs.. Breathe in & bring the hands up and repeat the twist to the right. Next movement involves turning the body to the left with your head and keeping eyes on the back of your heels. Repeat to the right side. Repeat this cycle 4 times.

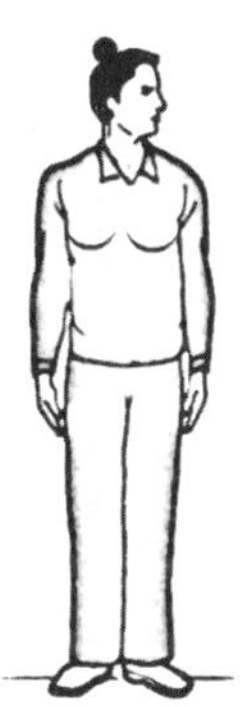 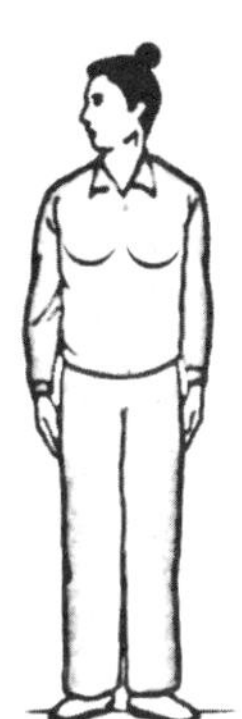 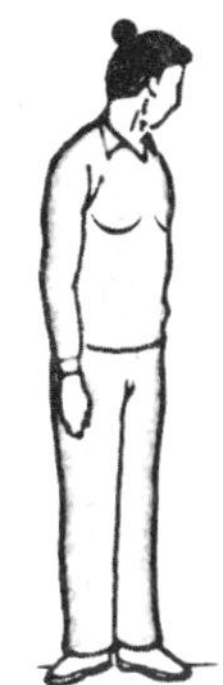

13. Lowering the Head and the Hips

Standing in attention with feet slightly apart and raise your right hand up in an arc above your head with the palm facing down. Breathe in and bend over to your left, letting your left arm hang loose to your left. Transfer all your body weight to the right leg, start breathing out and reach over the left to the furthest point that feels comfortable to you. Breathe in and straighten up with your right arm in an arch above your head. Breathe out as you lower your right arm. Breathe in and raise your left arm in an arch over your head and repeat the stretch. Next stand to attention with feet slightly apart and breathe in and raise your right hand up in arc above your head with the palm facing down, twist your upper torso to the left. Breathe out and bend to the left placing your left hand palm facing outward behind your back. Breathe in and stand to attention. Breathe in and straighten up with your left arm in an arch above your head, twist your upper torso to the right. Breathe out and bend to the right placing your right hand palm facing outward behind your back Repeat another round. Repeat this cycle 4 times.

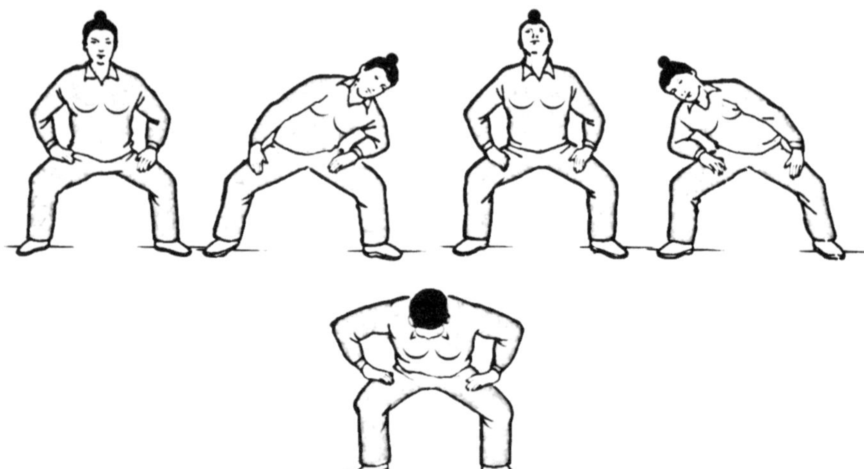

14. Touching the Toes with Both Hands

Standing to attention breathe in and raise both arms to the sides, palms facing up to shoulder level, then, up above your head. As you start to breathe out turn the palms face down and bring the arms down, outstretched behind you at shoulder level, downwards behind you, pulling your arms away from you and stretching for a few seconds. At this point each hand should be clasped together palms facing upward. Start to breathe in and release hands an straighten up slowly, bringing them up to your sides of your thighs. At this point you should be standing in attention again. Breathe in and raise both arms above your head hands facing each other. Breathe out and stretch and bend upper body forward, palms facing down. Imagine you want to touch the wall in front of you. As you continue down bend as far as possible and try to touch your toes. Breathe out and hold for a few seconds and then release. Breathe out bending your knees and roll your upper torso until you are standing straight. Breathe in and relax. Repeat another round. Repeat this cycle 4 times.

15. Clenching the Fist

Stand with legs wide apart bending the knees in a horse riding position and form a fist with each hand, folding your thumbs inside your fists. The elbows should be bent such that the fist are facing upend resting on each side of your waist. Breathe out slowly as you extend your left arm in front of you at shoulder level, turning the fist over to finish face down. Start to breathe in and as you pull your right elbow back, extend the right arms you did with the left. Continue to alternately breathe and extend the arms in this way for a minute. Rest and relax for a minute. Resume posture with legs wide apart and knees bent. This time drawing your left hand back thrust your right hand forward with force palm down. Draw right back and left hand fist forward with force. Repeat another round. Repeat this cycle 4 times.

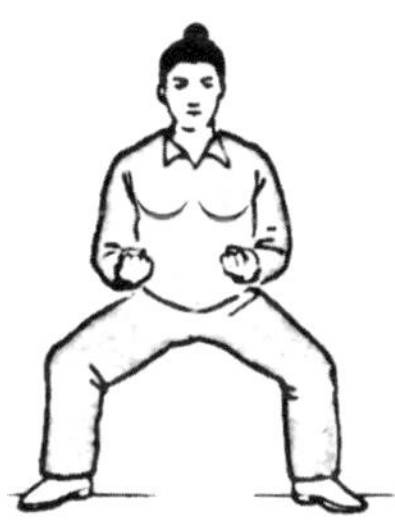
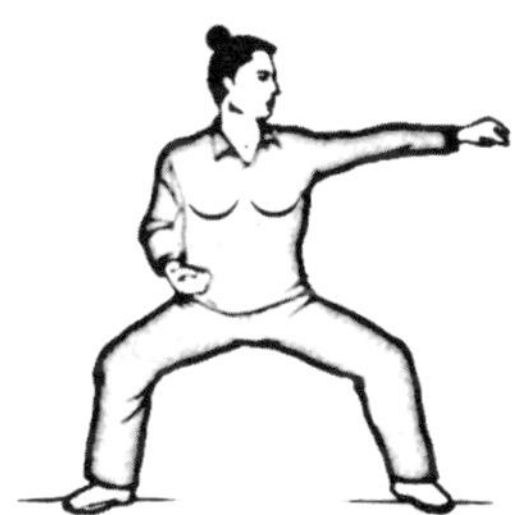

16. Shaking the Body

Bend knees to assume a horse riding position with legs wide apart, place hands on thighs, thumbs pointing upwards. Next, breathe in and place the backs of your hands on your lower back, closing your bowels. Shake your whole body by bouncing up and down gently, breathing out on each bounce. Next bend your upper body to left, swing head down and buttocks up to the right twice; keep left arm bent and right arm straight.. **Turn** head and upper body from right to front to **left.** Then come back and stand straight. This movement should be done in a continuous flow. Repeat another round. Repeat this cycle 4 times.

17. Heel Lifting

Stand to attention, hands behind your back, chest out, knees straight and legs together. Hold head up, left your heels as high as possible and breathe in. Breathe out and lower your heels slowly, but do not touch the ground. Breathe in and repeat it again for a few times, holding the heels off the ground for a few seconds more each new cycle. Breathe in slowly leaning forward, placing both hands flat on the floor, legs shoulder apart, bending your legs, if necessary. Breathe out slowly, aiming to straighten one leg, placing the heel down to the floor. Breathe repeating the stretch on the opposite leg, this time pushing down on your toes, with the heel raised slightly off the floor. Resting your hands on a raised platform will release the tension in the hamstrings. Repeat another round. Repeat this cycle 4 times.

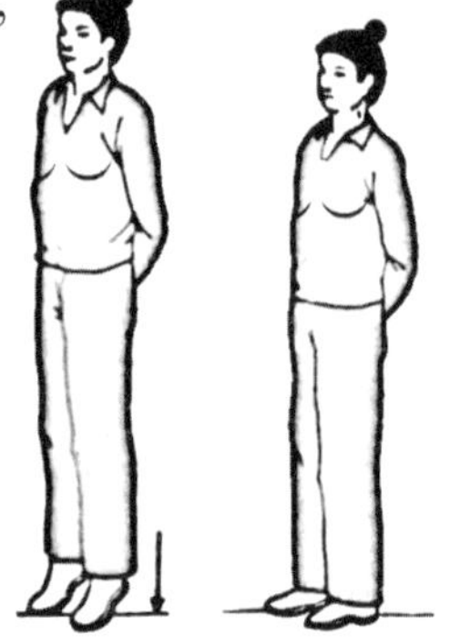

18. Horse Riding

Breathe in and bend knees and pretend that you are in a horse riding position. Lean forward, stretching your arms out in front of you, imagining you are holding the reins of the horse. Breathe out and in while at the same time lift and lower your heels in rapid succession and visualize yourself shaking your body as if you were riding a horse very fast. Do this for a few seconds. Breathe in and straighten knees and stand straight and breathe out. Repeat another round. Repeat this cycle 4 times.

System Three

19. Pressing the Heavens with Two Hands

Stand with feet shoulder width apart and arms hanging loosely on your side. Breathe in, head facing forward, open your legs shoulder apart and bend your knees and come into a horse riding position, with your hands resting on you thighs. Breathe out and raise your hands, fingers pointed out palms down, to the side of your head. Yours fingers should be facing your ears. Breathe in, bending forward and stretching your arms in front of you palms facing down, fingers touching until you touch the ground. If you don't touch the ground bed your knees until you do. Breathe out, and turn your palms facing upward, fingers touching, pushing your palms to the ground. Breathe in, turn your arms so that the palms face forward, clench your fists. While keeping your arms straight, imagine pulling up your body as if you were lifting a heavy weight. Breathe in, bend arms and lift fists to your chest. Breathe out, open your hands, palms down, moving your hands and arms upward and out, until you have formed a circle, keeping an eye on your finger tips. Breathe in, drop your hands to your side and bend your knees and come into the horse riding position. Breathe out and come into standing position with hands resting by your side. Repeat another round. Repeat this cycle 4 times.

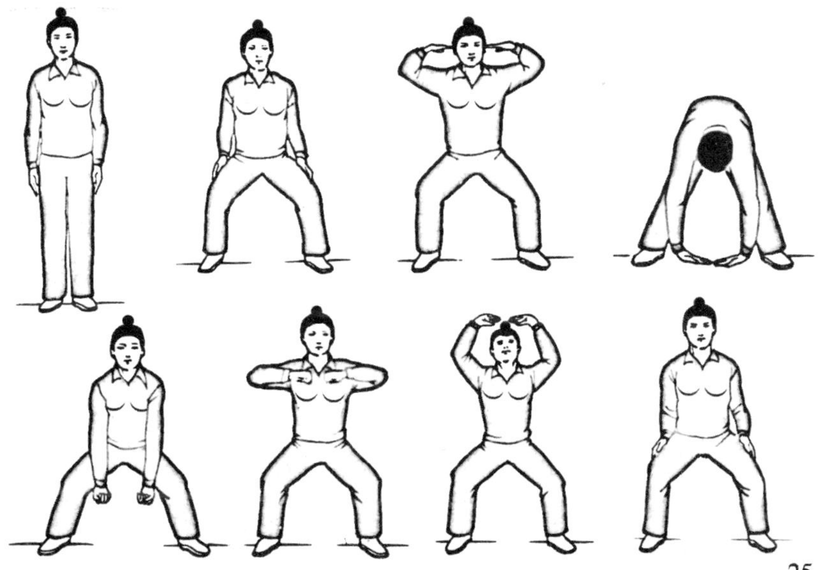

20. Drawing the Bow

Breathe in, turn your upper torso to the left, bend your knees and come into a horse riding position. Raise and bend your arms and clench your fists and hold your left hand at eye level and the right hand by your right shoulder. Keep your eyes on the left fist. Breathe out, stretch your right arm to the right and pull your left elbow to the left until both fists are at shoulder level. Turn your head to look at your left fist and then at your right. Breathe in, turning your head to the right shoulder at eye level. Keep your eyes on the right fist. Breathe out, stretch your left arm to the left and pull your left elbow to the left until both fists are at shoulder level. Repeat another round. Repeat this cycle 4 times.

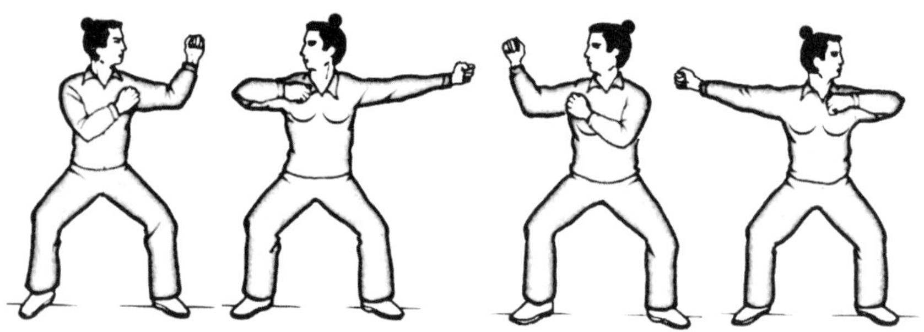

21. Holding up a Single Hand

Stand straight, feet shoulder apart, arms by your sides and come into a horse riding position. Breathe in, turning your body to the right straightening your left leg out, with your right leg bent. Bring your hands into a fist position and hold your left fist pointing upwards to eye level and your right fist pointing forward near your waist, keeping your eyes on the left fist. Breathe out, bending forward unclench your fists, pushing your left palm down to touch your left foot. Keep your right hand at your waist, palm up, with your eyes on left hand. Breathe in, turning your upper torso to the left, keeping your right leg straight, bend your left knee, and bend your left arm back toward your face so that your fingers point at your nose and eyes. Breathe out, pushing your left hand, palm up; while pressing down with your right hand, palm down. Keep your eyes on the left hand. Repeat this movement but in the opposite direction. Breathe in, turning your body to the left straightening your right leg out, with your left leg bent. Bring your hands into a fist position and hold your right fist pointing upwards to eye level and your left fist pointing forward near your waist, keeping your eyes on the right fist. Breathe out, bending forward unclench your fists, pushing your right palm down to touch your right foot. Keep your left hand at your waist, palm up, with your eyes on right hand. Breathe in, turning your upper torso to the right, keeping your left leg straight, bend your right knee, and bend your right arm back toward your face so that your fingers point at your nose and eyes. Breathe out, pushing your right hand, palm up; while pressing down with your left hand, palm down. Keep your eyes on the right hand. Repeat another round. Repeat this cycle 4 times.

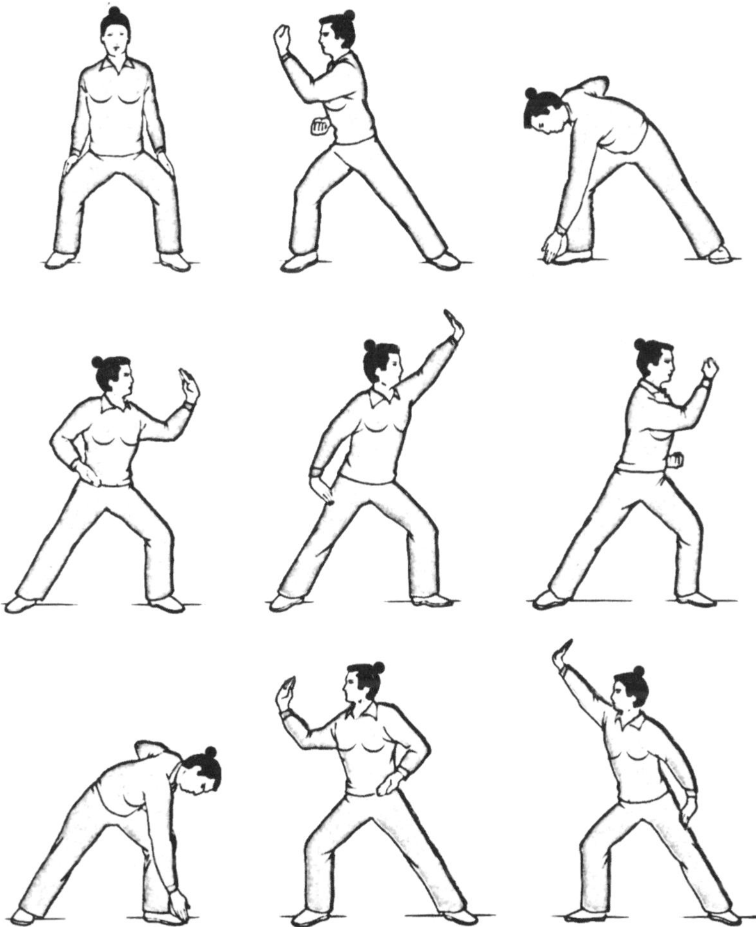

22. Looking back Like a Cow Gazing at the Moon

Stand to attention, separate legs shoulder width and come into a horse riding position. Breath in, hold your hands in clenched fists with your right fist at chest level and your left fist at stomach level with your left fist closer to your body. Breathe out, turning your body to the left, keeping your right leg straight, and bending your left knee. At the same time unclench your sits and pushing up with your right hand, fingers pointing upward, and your left hand towards the ground, fingers pointing down, turning your head backward looking over your left shoulder. Breathe in, turning your body back to center, back straight and in horse riding position.. Breath in, hold your hands in clenched fists with your right fist at chest level and your right fist at stomach level with your right fist closer to your body. Breathe out, turning your body to the right, keeping your left leg straight, and bending your right knee. At the same time unclench your sits and pushing up with your left hand, fingers pointing upward, and your right hand towards the ground, fingers pointing down; turn your head backward looking over your right shoulder. Breathe in, turning your body back to center, back straight and in horse riding position. Repeat another round. Repeat this cycle 4 times.

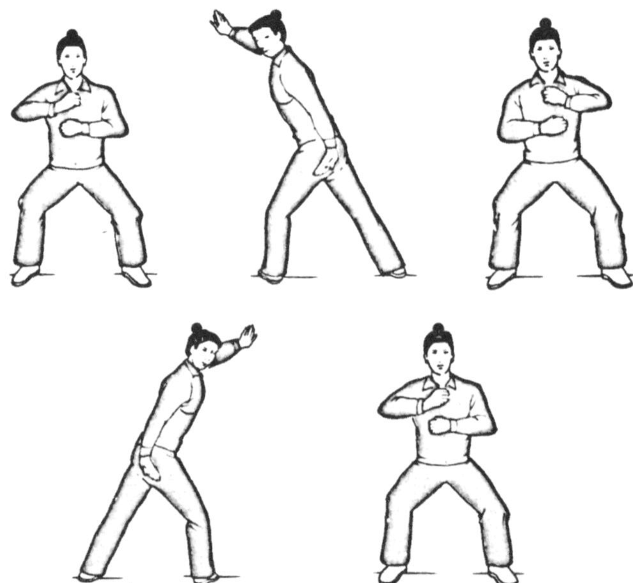

23. Lowering the Head and the Hips

Standing in attention with feet slightly apart and shoulder width apart, place your hands on your waist, palms up, and looking straight of you. Breathe in, stretching both hands forward, bend your waist without curving your back, and bring hands down to the ground and touch your toes, looking straight ahead of you. Breathe out, stretch your hands out bringing both hands out until you are in standing position again. Breathe in, stretching both hands forward, bending your waist without curving your back, and bring your hands down to the ground and touch your toes, looking straight ahead of you, and turn your head to the right. Breathe out; stretch your hands out bringing both hands out until you are in standing position again. Breathe in, stretching both hands forward, bend your waist without curving your back, and bring hands down to the ground and touch your toes, looking straight ahead of you and turn your head to the left. Breathe out; stretch your hands out bringing both hands out until you are in standing position again. Repeat another round. Repeat this cycle 4 times.

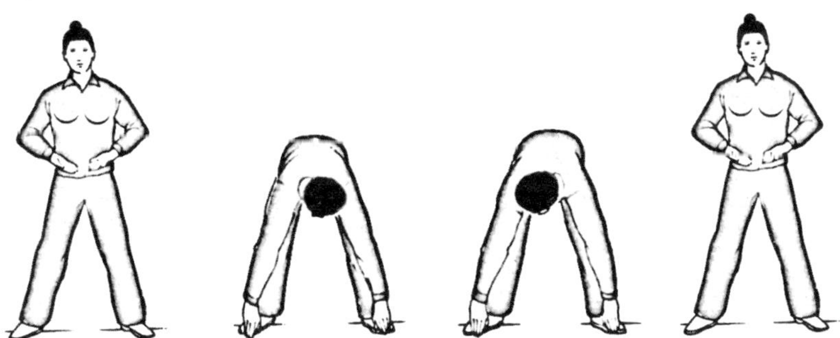

24. Touching the Toes

Come to a standing attention with your legs straight, breathe in and raise your left leg and stretch out your arms and hold both toes with both of your hands and look straight ahead. Breathe out and come back to standing attention. Breathe in, and raise your right leg up and stretch both arms out and grab both toes with both hands. Breathe out and come back to standing attention. Repeat another round. Repeat this cycle 4 times.

25. Fist Playing with Eyes Glaring

Come into standing position, and breathe in, bending your knees place put yourself in the horse riding position.forming a fist with each hand, folding your thumbs inside your fists. The elbows should be bent such that the fist are facing upend resting on each side of your waist. Breathe out slowly as you extend your left arm in front of you at shoulder level, turning the fist over to finish face down. Looking straight ahead at a point in front of you breathe in and out a few times, keeping your posture strong and firm. Breathe in, and come back to standing position and relax with hands to yo9ur side. Repeat this cycle 4 times.

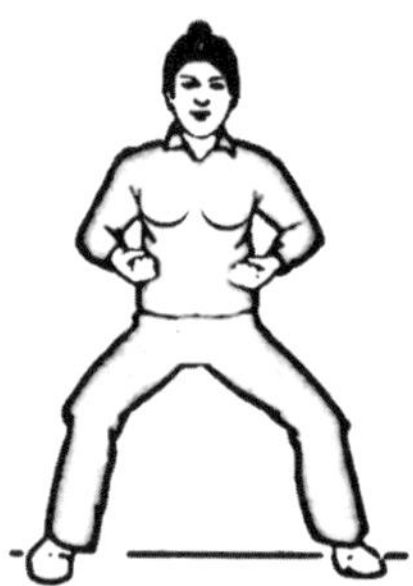

26. Shaking the Body

Bend knees to assume a horse riding position with legs wide apart, place hands on thighs, thumbs pointing upwards. Next, breathe in and place the backs of your hands on your lower back, closing your bowels. Shake your whole body by bouncing up and down gently, breathing out on each bounce. Next bend your upper body to left, swing head down and buttocks up to the right twice; keep left arm bent and right arm straight.. Turn head and upper body from right to front to left. Then come back and stand straight. This movement should be done in a continuous flow. Repeat this cycle 4 times.

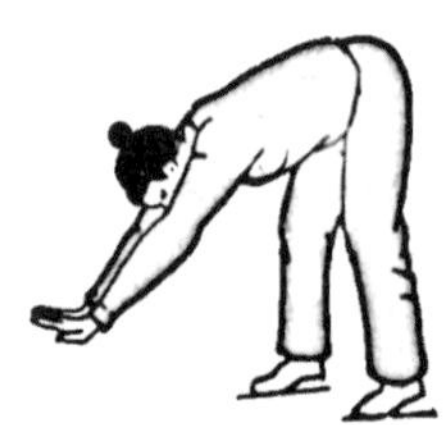

27. Heel Lifting

Stand to attention, hands behind to your side. Breathe in and raise both hands to the air arms and hands facing each other, fingers pointing to the sky. Shift the weight of your body to the balls of your feet and raise your heels up and hold for a second. Breathe out and lower your heels down but do not touch the ground. Keeping your arms and hands in the air breathe in, and raise your heels up for a second and breathe out lowering your heels with out touching the ground. Repeat this cycle 4 times.

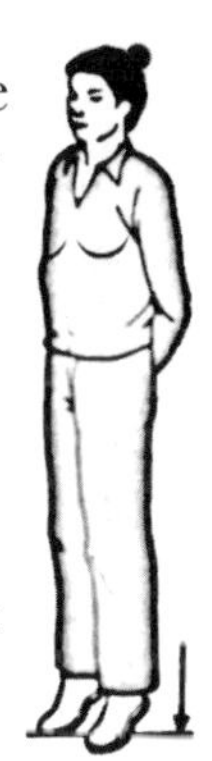

System Four

The following exercises are to be done in a sitting posture. It is recommended doing them before you go to work in the morning and/or before you go to bed in the evening.

28 Hugging the Head

Sit on the floor in a half-lotus position. Sitting in **half-**lotus position requires one foot be crossed over **onto** the thigh of the other. The other foot will be placed underneath the raised leg. Hold your hands **if** front of abdomen, breathing normally and focus on the abdominal area. Breathe in, bringing both your hands fingers interlocked, behind your head. Breathe out, and look; pressing your hands forward, breathe in, looking down. Repeat a number of times. Breathe in, and turn your head to the left, and press your hands to the right, breathe out, turning to the opposite direction. Do this several times. Allow your eyes to follow as your head turns in each direction. Repeat a number of times. This exercise strengthens your neck muscles and allows more blood to circulate in the neck and head.

29 Rolling the Head

Sit on the floor in a cross legged half-lotus position. Relax your shoulders and your head, resting your hands on your knees try not to move your shoulders and your arms as you roll your head from side to side. Breathe in, rolling your head in a half arc from the right, breathe out rolling your head to the left. Do this a few times. Try to contract and expand your abdominal area as you roll your head. Your neck muscles should also be relaxed as you roll your head. This exercise relieves tension tense in the neck and shoulder area and generally relaxes the upper torso. Repeat this cycle 4 times.

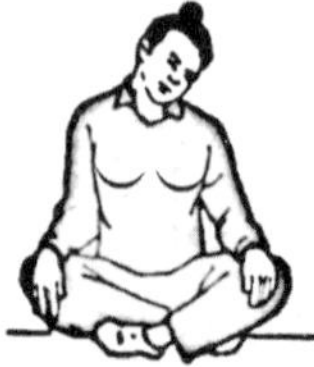
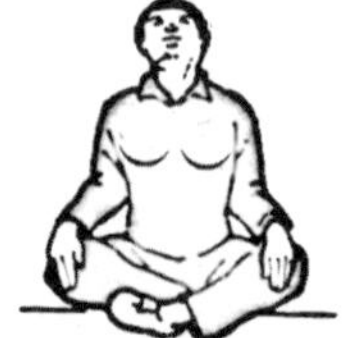
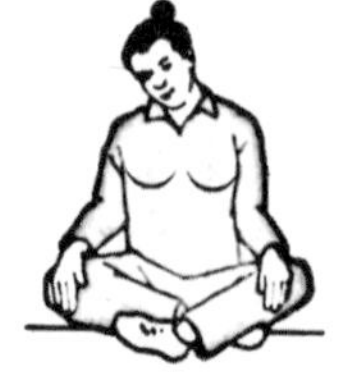

30 Holding your Hands to the Heavens

Sit on the floor in a half lotus position and breathe in, raise your hands over head with your fingers interlocked, turning your palms over and stretching them upwards. Make sure your arms are extended and elbows are straight with your adnominal muscles pulled in. Breathe out, and relax your hands on top of your head. This movement will strengthen your arm, hands and shoulder muscles. Repeat this cycle 4 times.

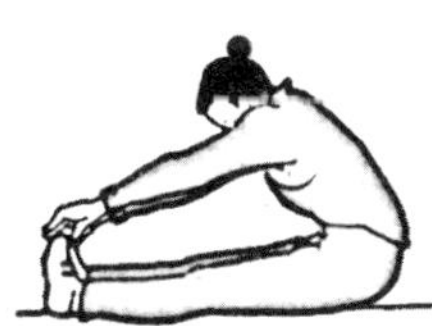

31 Reaching for your toes

Sit on the floor with your palms lightly touching your thighs. Lift your arms to chest level, palms facing out. Breathe in, bend forward as far as possible, keeping your back straight, knees together, legs straight, extend your arms out in front of you and grab hold of your toes or touch your toes. Remember to keep your back and arms straight and bring your forehead as close to knees as possible. Breathe out, and let go of toes and come back to a sitting position with your palms resting on your thighs and your back straight. This movement strengthens your lower back, abdominal area, and leg muscles. Repeat this cycle 4 times.

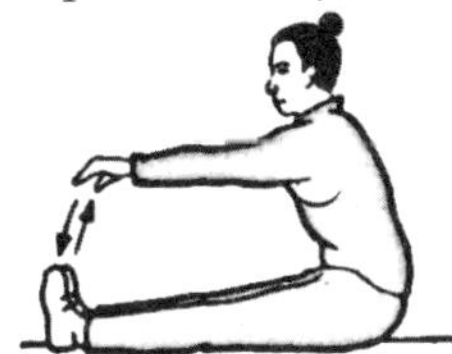

32 Wheeling your arms

Sitting with your legs straight breathe in, extend your arms in front of you at chest level, with your fists extended out move them downward toward your knees and up to your chest. Breathe out, and move your fists up extend your arms and bring your

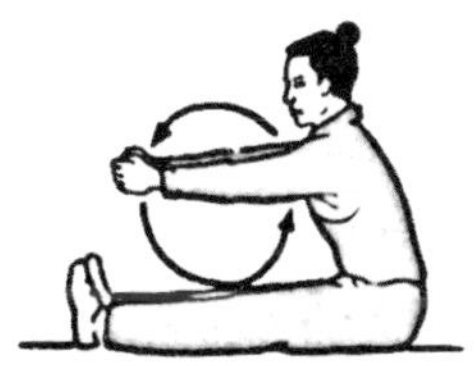

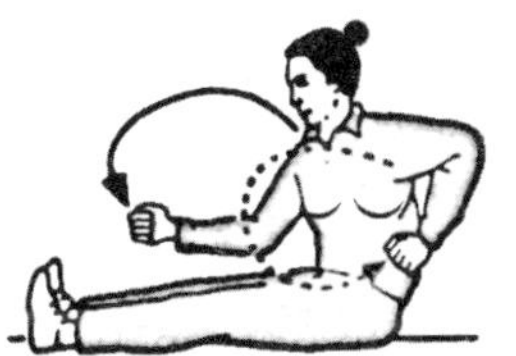

fists back in front of you. Repeat this wheel like motion in the opposite direction. Breathe in, moving your extended fists upward to your chest. Breathe out, bringing your fists down toward your knees and back up to chest level in front of you. Keeping your arms extended out in front of you with fists facing away from you, breathe in, keeping your right fist in front of you, bend your left elbow and bring your left fist to the side of your waist. Breathe out, bring your left fist back in front of you while you bend the right elbow and bring your right fist to the side of your waist. Move your head and shoulders as you alternative each fist going back and forth. Repeat this cycle 4 times.

33 Drawing the Bow

Sit in a half-lotus position, breath in, turn your head to the right, bring your hands up to your chest extending your right hand, forefinger, and middle finger, pointing up to the right, keeping your eyes following your fingers. Bend your left elbow and bring your left hand to shoulder level near your chest and imagine you are pulling on a bow. Breathe out, releasing your arms and hands, turn your head back to center and rest your hands on your knees. Breathe in turn your head to the left, bring your hands up to your chest extending your left hand, forefinger, and middle finger, pointing up to the left, keeping your eyes following your fingers. Bend your right elbow and bring your right hand to shoulder level near your chest and imagine you are pulling on a bow. Breathe out, releasing your arms and hands, turn your head back to center and rest your hands on your knees. This motion increases your lung capacity, and strengthens your back and arms muscles. Repeat this cycle 4 times.

34 Crisscross Fist Play

Sit in a half-lotus position, hands resting on your knees, breathe in, raise your left arm to shoulder level, jab your left arm out away from your body, hand clenched fist facing away from you, right hand with fist facing away from you resting on your right thigh.

Breathe out, raising your right fist to shoulder level, thrust your right fist out in front you, while you bringing the left arm down to rest on your left thigh. Hands resting on your knees breathe in, raise your left arm to shoulder level, jab your left arm out away from your body to the right side of your body, hand clenched fist facing away from you, right hand with fist facing away from you resting on your right thigh. Breathe out, raising your right fist to shoulder level, jab your right fist out in front you to the left side of your body, while you bringing your right arm down to rest on your left thigh. Repeat this cycle a number of times. This movement strengthens your arms and shoulder muscles.

Repeat this cycle 4 times.

35 Hitting the Whole Body

Sitting in half-lotus, breathing normally, clench hands into a fist position and begin lightly hitting your body with both fists, beginning on your knees, thighs, stomach, chest, back, shoulders, neck, arms, and top of your head. This stimulate and relaxes your muscles as if someone is giving you massage. Repeat this cycle 4 times rest for a couple of minutes and repeat cycle 4 times.

Baby and Child Workouts

Exercise for infants (Static and Inter-Active Exercises) basically involves playful yet purposeful interaction. Infants need to see new sights; to be touched; to wiggle and explore; to move their body parts; and to reach and grasp out into their new world. Advanced educational degrees, expensive toys, and state-of-the-art equipment are not necessary to support healthy infant development. However, love, gentle caresses, and regular communication are priceless. Here are three set of exercises for babies between 2 months and one and half years old. Remember that regularity and promptness in exercising baby workouts are essential.

Child workouts for two and three year olds occurs at a time when they are learning to master basic movements like walking, running, kicking, and throwing. Kids this age are naturally active, so give your child lots of opportunities to practice and build on these skills. By encouraging your child to engage in active play, you are helping your child to be physically fit now and in the future.

Static Exercises for Babies
System One

Here are 8 simple interactions and "exercise routines" you can perform with the infants two and six month old babies to assist in their mental and physical development. Babies 2 and 4 month should only perform the first exercises and the last one. Babies between 4 and 6 months should do all 8 exercises.

If you find your baby is resistant to any of these exercises do not force them to do them.

Chest Movement Number 1- Prepare your baby by placing him/her on a comfortable bed or table. Start by talking gently and rubbing his/her chest down to their abdomen. Then take the baby's arms and make sure the arms are straight. Have the baby grab your thumbs. Next spread your baby's arms side to side with its palms facing up and bring the baby's arms in and across their chest and gently press their abdomen. Repeat each cycle 4 times with a rest period between each cycle.

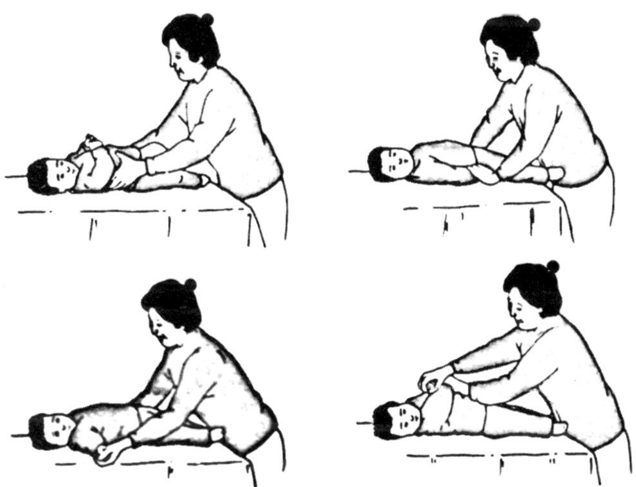

Extending Arms Prepare baby as in # 1. Take your babies hands and pull them up facing each other and then stretch the hands above the head shoulder length apart. It is important to remember to be gentle while exercising with your baby. Repeat each cycle 4 times with a rest period between each cycle.

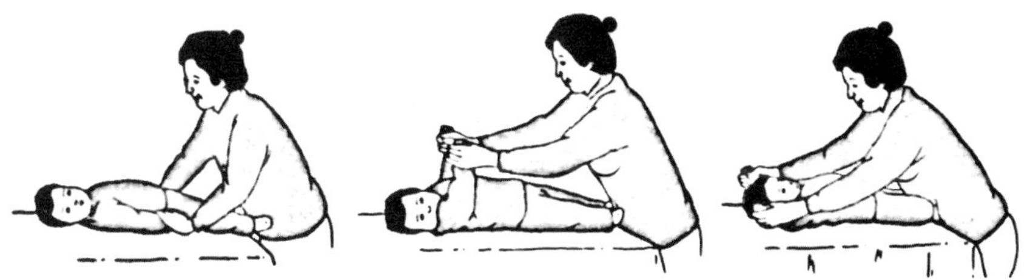

Bending Legs – Prepare baby as in # 1. Holding your baby's legs bend their knees toward their chest and then straight then out by pulling them back towards you. Repeat each cycle 4 times with a rest period between each cycle.

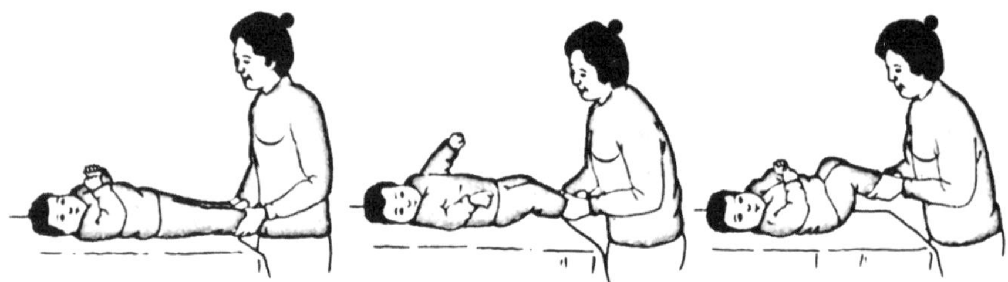

Lifting Legs – Prepare baby as in #1. Hold on to your babies legs raise them up at a 90-degree angle keeping their lower back on the ground. Repeat each cycle 4 times with a rest period between each cycle.

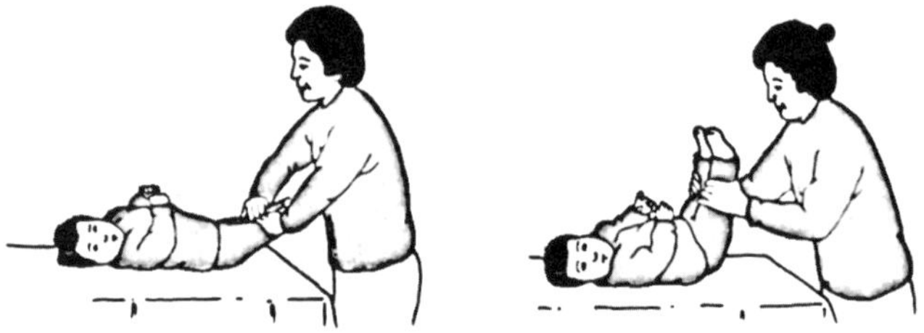

Revolving Shoulders – Prepare baby as in # 1. Holding your babies hands slowly and gently stretch the arms outward rotating away form his/her chest. Return hands to center. Holding your baby's hands stretch and rotate the baby's arms inward from the chest. Repeat each cycle 4 times with a rest period between each cycle.

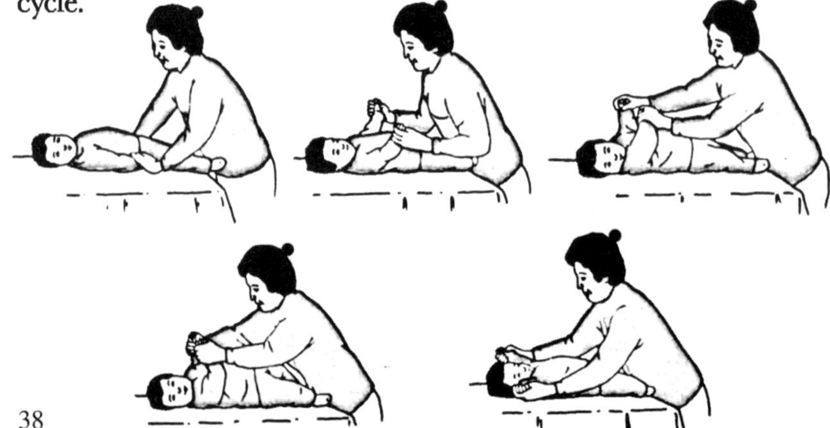

Arching Back – Place your baby on their stomach with their arms facing away from their body. Holding both legs gently left the legs keeping their stomach on the ground. Slowly return their legs to the ground. Hold onto the babies elbows and raise their upper torso off the ground keeping their abdomen on the ground. Gently lower the baby back to the ground. Repeat each cycle 4 times with a rest period between each cycle.

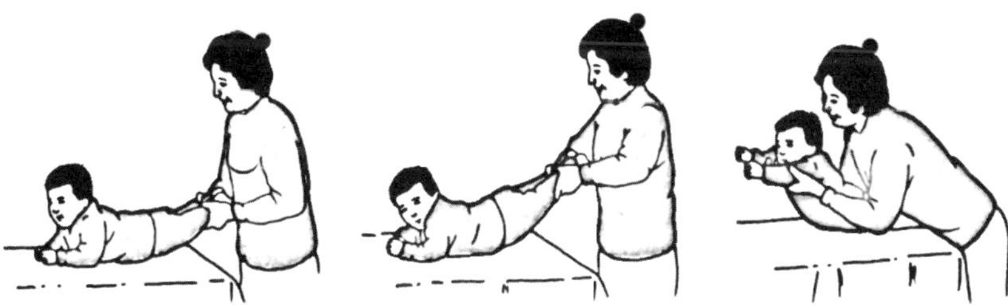

Rotating – Prepare baby as in # 1. Turn your baby on their right side and hold on to their right arm and right leg at the same time and gently pull them up together, then returning them to their body. Rotate your baby to their left side and lift the left arm and left leg at the same time and then return them to their body. Repeat each cycle 4 times with a rest period between each cycle.

Relaxing – Gentle rub you're your babies arms, legs, stomach and let them lie down in an in-active state for a few minutes to relax. Depending on the nature and temperament of your baby you could repeat the whole series again.

Inter-Active Exercises
System Two

These exercises are for six to 1 year old babies. Babies between 6 to 9 months should only do the first 5 exercises, whereas babies between 9 to 12 months may do all 9 sets.

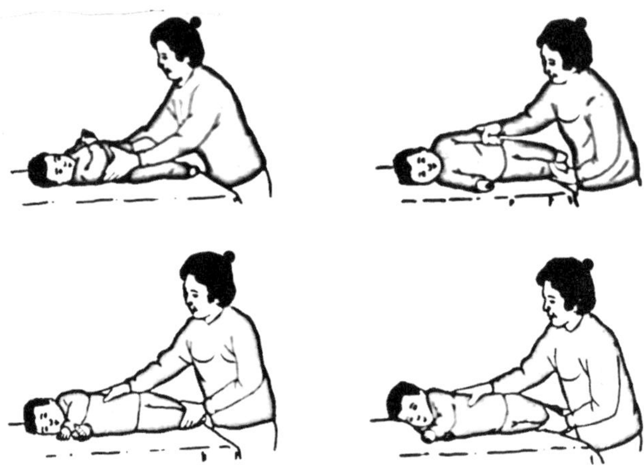

Chest Movement - Prepare your baby by placing him/her on a comfortable bed or table. Start by talking gently and rubbing his/her chest down to their abdomen. Then take the baby's arms and make sure the arms are straight. Have the baby grab your thumbs. Next spread your baby's arms side to side with its palms facing up and bring the baby's arms in and across their chest and gently press their abdomen. Repeat each cycle 4 times with a rest period between each cycle.

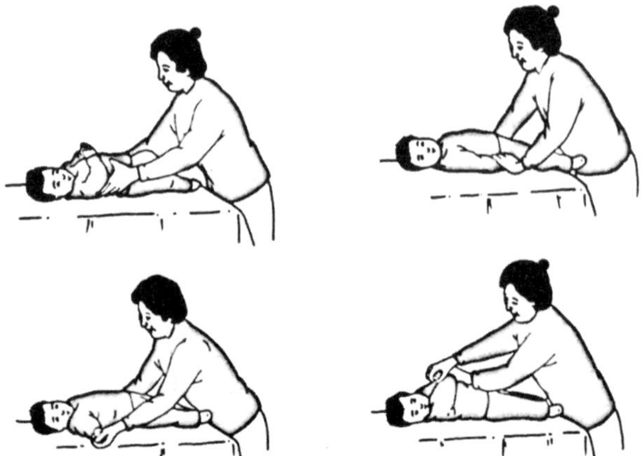

Extending Arms – Prepare your baby as in # 1. Take your babies hands and pull them up facing each other and then stretch the hands above the head shoulder length apart. It is important to remember to be gentle while exercising with your baby. Repeat each cycle 4 times with a rest period between each cycle.

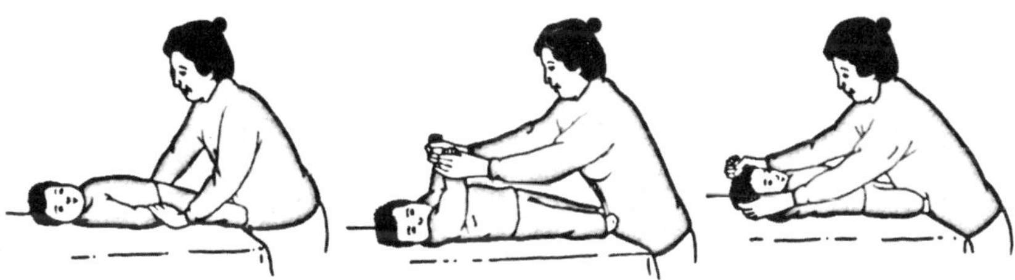

Bending Legs – Prepare your baby as in #1. Holding your baby's legs bend their left knee toward their chest making sure to keep his right leg straight. While bringing his left back bend his right knee. Do this three of four times. Repeat each cycle 4 times with a rest period between each cycle. Repeat each cycle 4 times with a rest period between each cycle.

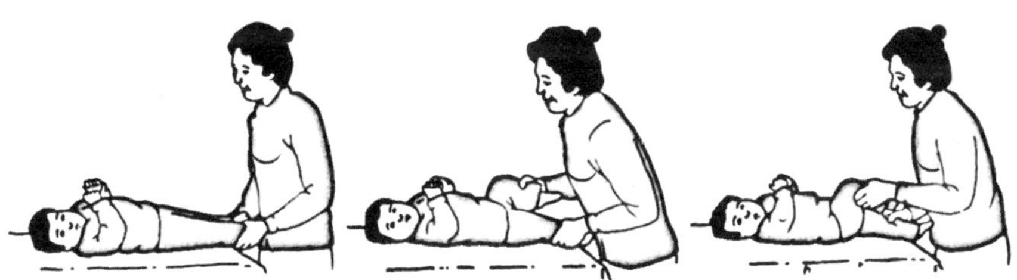

Sitting Up – Have your baby lie on their back. Gently hold on their hands and pull them up into a sitting position. Then slowly let the baby roll back into a lying position. A Variation for six to 9 month old babies is to allow them to stand up from their sitting position. Remembering to be gentle and careful not to be to quick when going from sitting to standing. Repeat each cycle 4 times with a rest period between each cycle.

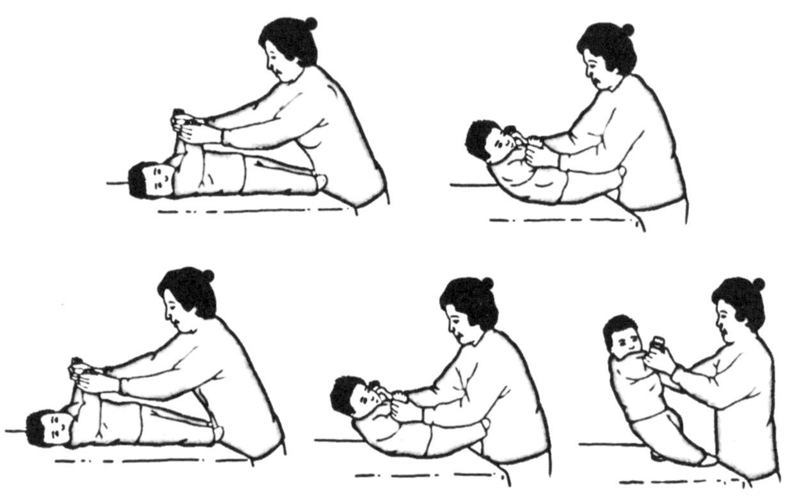

Bending Down and Standing Up – Hold on to your babies arms and gently pull them up into a standing position. Stand behind your baby and firmly wrap your arms around the babies' waist and let them bend forward to grab something they like to play with. Once they grab it bring them back slowly to standing position. Repeat each cycle 4 times with a rest period between each cycle.

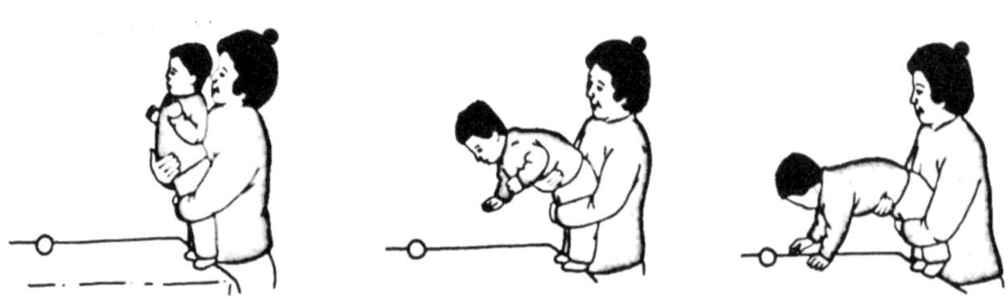

Rising and Crouch – Stand in front of your baby and grab your babies arms, gently raising your baby into a standing position. Grab your baby under their arms. Gently lower the baby down in a crouching position. Repeat each cycle 4 times with a rest period between each cycle.

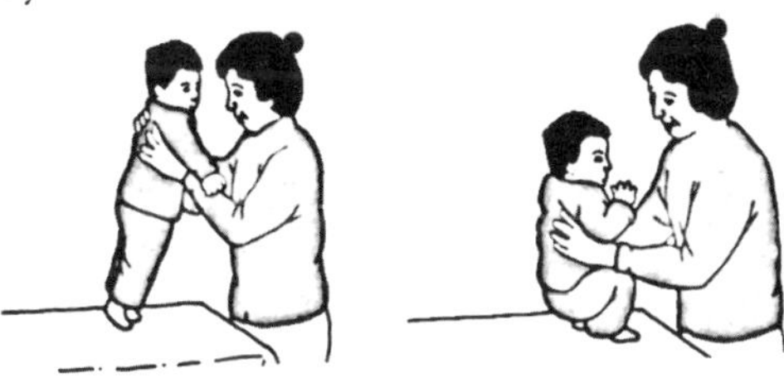

Jumping – Stand in front of your baby and grab your babies' arms and gently stand him/her up. Placing your hands under their arms lift the baby up and encourage your baby to jump up. Repeat each cycle 4 times with a rest period between each cycle.

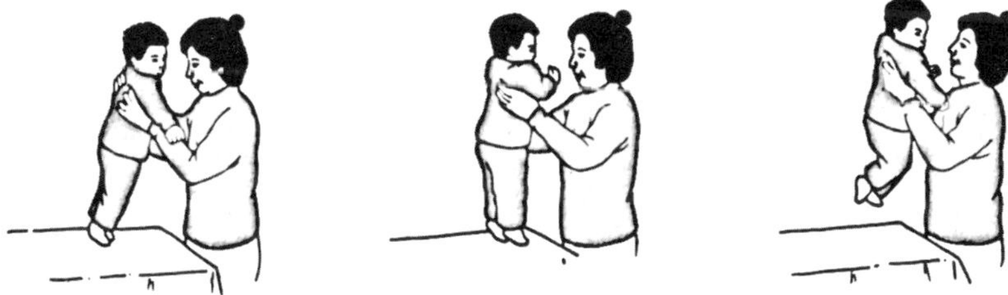

Relaxing – Gentle rub you're your babies' arms, legs, stomach and let them lie down in an in-active state for a few minutes to relax. Depending on the nature and temperament of your baby you could repeat the whole series again.

Double Pole Exercises
System Three

The following exercises are children one and half to 2 years old. Use two one metre long bamboo poles or of broom sticks with the broom cut off or two plastic poles. Make sure they are thin enough for your child to hold on too. You will need two people (adults) to assist with this exercise.

Arm Rolling – Have two adults sit on small chairs or stools (make sure the height of the chairs are waist height of your child) facing each other, holding both ends of the poles. Your child should stand in the middle of these poles and hold on to sides of the poles. Each adult moves the poles alternately backwards and forwards gently and rhythmically, so that your child's arms swing repeatedly with the poles. Repeat this 4 times with a rest period between each.

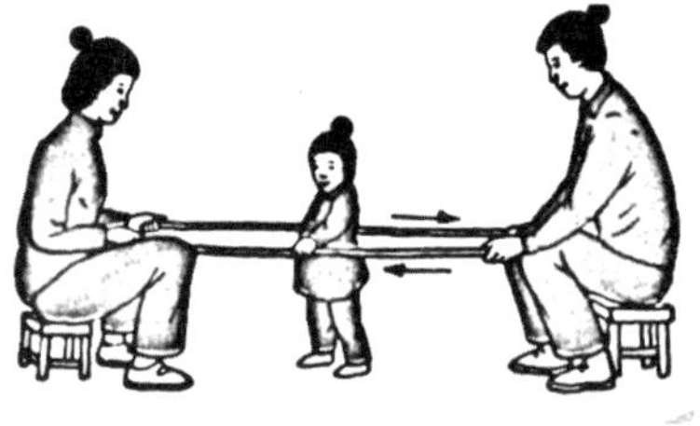

Stretching – Preparation as in # 1. Move the poles horizontally so your child's arms are stretched out to the side. Raise the poles in the air so that your child's arms are raised over their head. Bring the poles back down so your child's arms are stretched out to the side. Bring the poles back to center and have child relax. Be aware during this exercise that the child's arms are not stretched too far or for too long. Repeat each cycle 4 times with a rest period between each cycle.

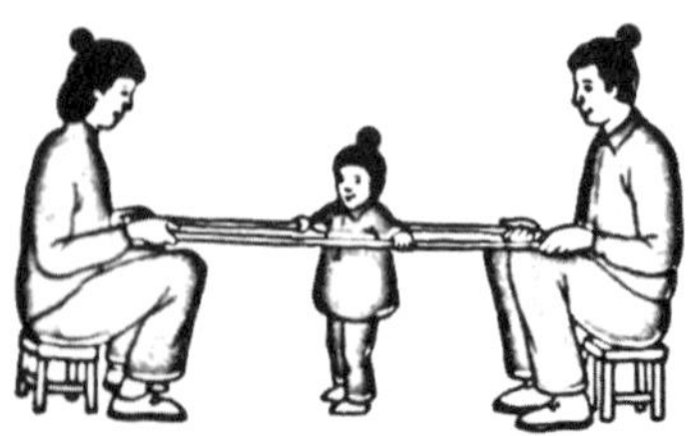

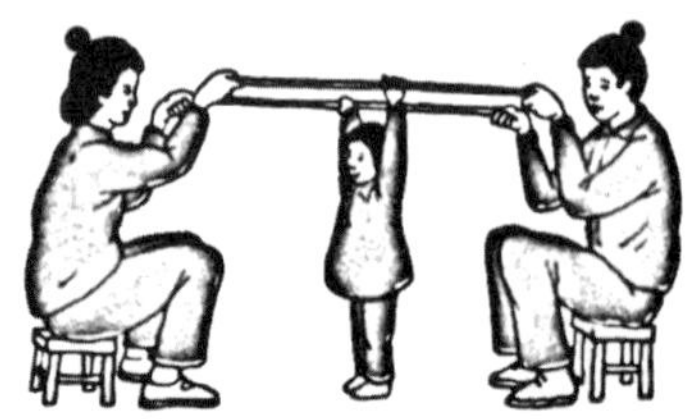

Twisting Sideways – Preparation as in # 1. Have child grip the poles. Adults move the poles sideways so your child's arms are stretched. The person behind your child moves the pole up above its head and the person facing your child moves the pole toward them so that your child will be stretched and twisted at the same time. The person in front of your child moves the pole above its head and the person behind your child moves the pole backwards towards them. Your child is stretched and twisted in a different direction. Try to keep your child's legs straight and while twisting your child make sure you are gentle. Repeat each cycle 4 times with a rest period between each cycle.

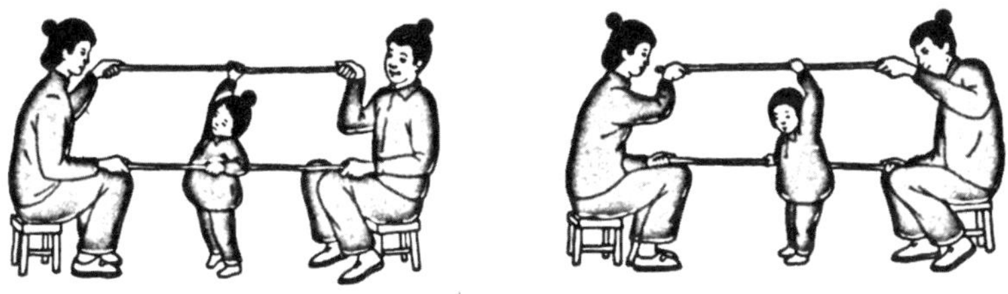

Crouching – Preparation as in # 1. Move the poles horizontally so your child's arms are stretched out to the side. Slowly lower the poles down encouraging your child to bend their knees as the pole is lowered closer to the ground. Once your child is in crouching or in a squatting position begin raising the poles up again so that your child is standing straight.. Move the poles horizontally so your child's arms are stretched out again to the side. Bring the poles back to center and have child relax. Repeat each cycle 4 times with a rest period between each cycle.

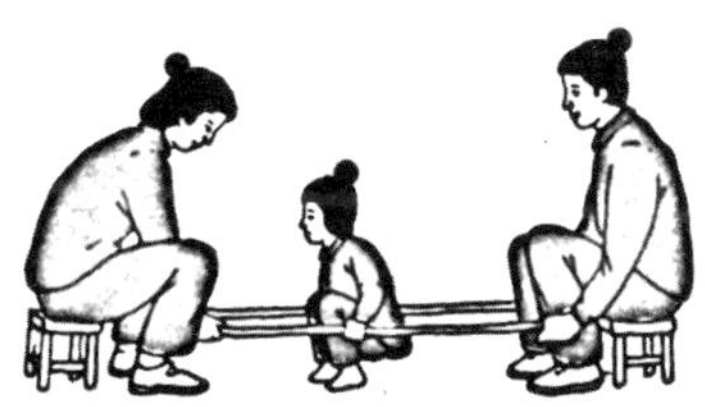

Stepping Forward and Backward – Preparation as in # 1. Move the poles backward and forward while the child grips the poles and is encouraged to try walk backwards and forward. Be aware of your child's balance and be gentle. Repeat each cycle 4 times with a rest period between each cycle.

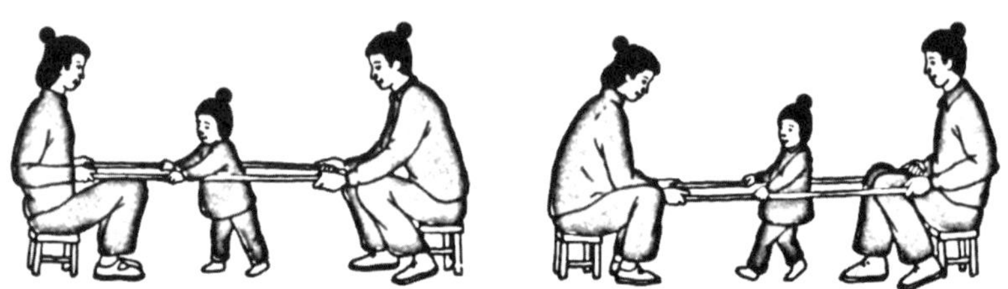

Hanging and Swinging – Preparation as in # 1. Move the poles horizontally so your child's arms are stretched out to the side. Raise the poles in the air so that your child's arms are raised over their head. Carefully, raise the pole that your child's feet are off the ground. Encourage your child to swing back and forth and side to side. Slowly lower your child back to the ground. Bring the poles back down so your child's arms are stretched out to the side. Bring the poles back to center and have child relax. Be aware during this exercise that the child's arms are not stretched too far or high for too long. Repeat each cycle 4 times with a rest period between each cycle.

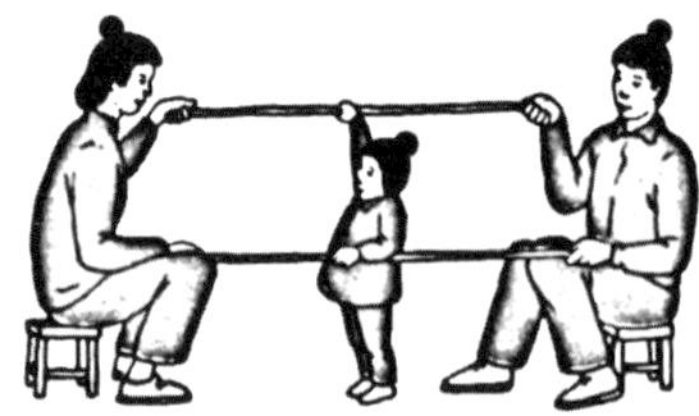

Jumping – Preparation as in # 1. Bring the pole under your child's arms. Make sure your child grips the poles and carefully lift your child off the ground. Encourage your child to jump up and down as you gently raise and lower the poles. Carefully lower your child back to the ground. Repeat each cycle 4 times with a rest period between each cycle.

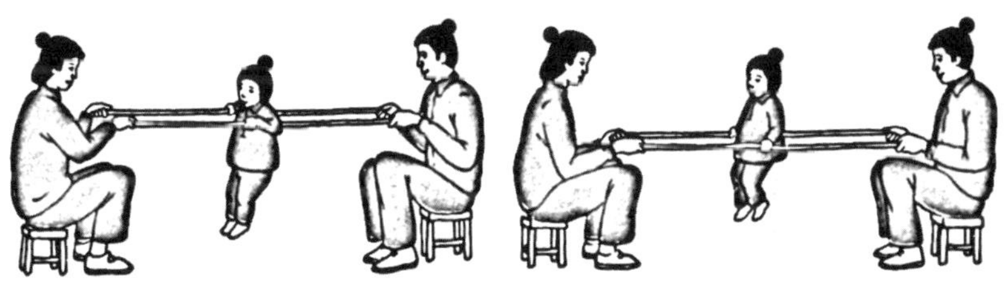

Skipping – Preparation as in # 1. Bring the pole under your child's arms. Make sure your child grips the poles and carefully lift your child off the ground. Encourage your child to skip as you gently raise and lower the poles. Carefully lower your child back to the ground. Repeat each cycle 4 times with a rest period between each cycle.

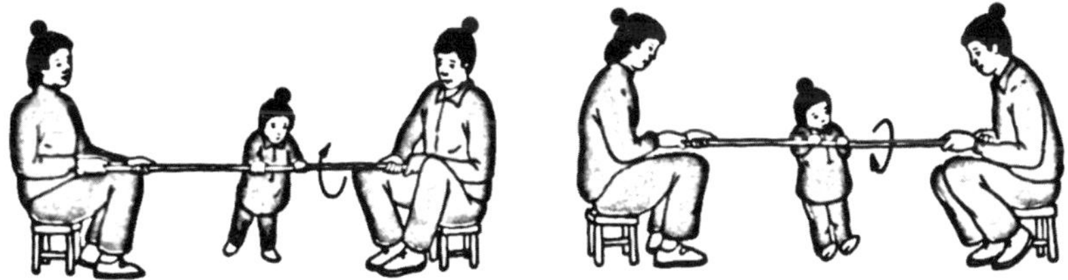

Fitness Workouts for any Purpose

These series of exercises were developed from the traditional movements of Wushu for fitness workouts for any purpose that can be done at home or at work. They are divided into 3 sections; Home Movements, Office Movements and Fifteen Minute Break Movements. Each section is divided into a series of postures and exercises to help relieve the stress from daily life

Home Movements – Section One
Set One

Breathe in, stand with your feet together, legs straight, arms slightly bent to your side, chest out and stomach in. Breathe out; slowly raising your hands in a criss-cross position in front of your chest until your hands are above your head. Stretch them to the side of your body with your hands hooked down and wrists higher than your shoulders. Breathe in, lowering your arms and push straight forward from waist level with open hands, palms facing each other with your arms shoulder-level high and shoulder-width apart. Breathe out, bringing your hands back to your waist with stretch arms, first to the side and then to the front of you. Clench your fists and bend elbows at shoulder level. Breathe in, returning to a standing position with your arms resting to your sides. Repeat this cycle 4 times.

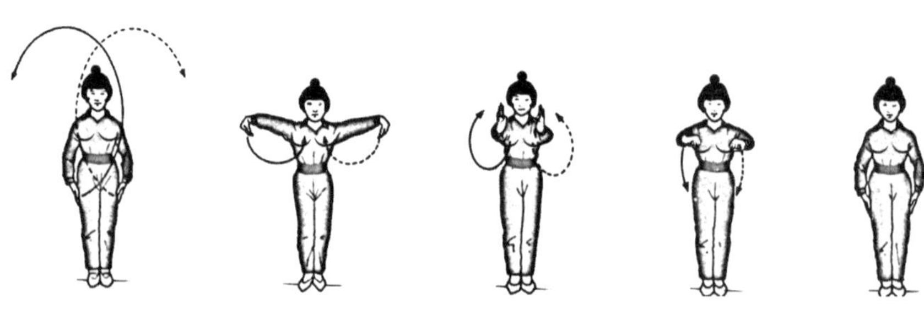

Breathe in, stand with your feet together, legs straight, arms slightly bent to your side, chest out and stomach in. Breathe out; with your hands at your waist step to the left, keeping your right leg straight, bending your left leg, and turning your body to the left. Breathe in, pushing away from your body with open palms, with arms at shoulder level. Putting weight on your right foot turn your body toward the right, bringing your left foot in, keeping your toes to the ground, while at the same time bring your arms in at chest level and press down with clenched fists. Breathe out, come back into standing position. Repeat in the opposite direction. Repeat this cycle 4 times.

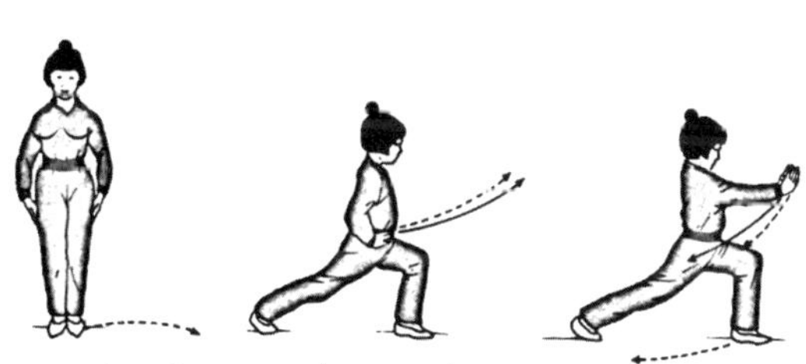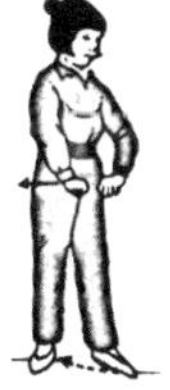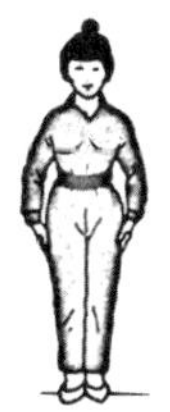

Breathe in, stand with your feet together, legs straight, arms slightly bent to your side, chest out and stomach in. Breathe out, stepping to your left, keeping your toes close to the ground. Bend knees to assume a horse-riding position, chest out, stomach in, and in a continuous motion cross arms in front, lift them above head, stretch them to the side in a curve and return them to waist with clenched fists, palms up. Breathe out, turning to your left, keep your right leg straight, and bend your left leg, Thrust right fist forward with palm down. Breathe in, turning to your right, return to the horse-riding position. At the same time lift right arm up and thrust left fist to the left. Breathe out, return to standing position. Repeat this in the opposite direction. Repeat this cycle 4 times.

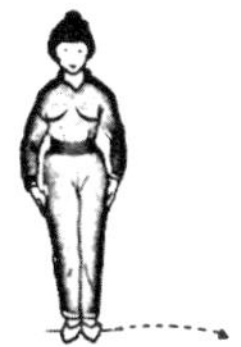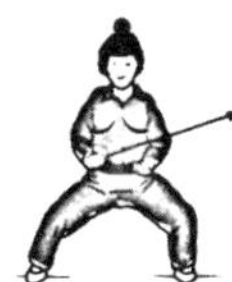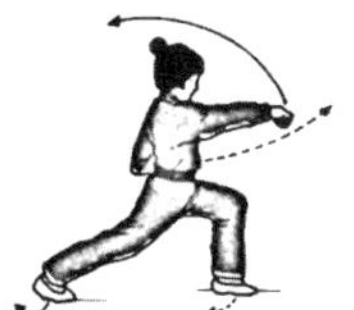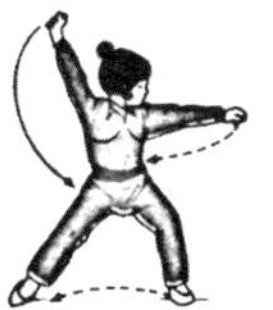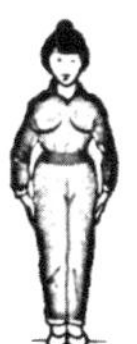

Breathe in, stand with your feet together, legs straight, arms slightly bent to your side, chest out and stomach in. Breathe out, lift your right fist straight up above your head, while keeping your left fist at your waist, with your palm up and turn to the left. Breathe in, leap to your left, following with your right foot, lift your right heel off the ground and bend both your knees slightly. At the same time raise your left arm, palm up, and lower your right arm, pressing down your fist (fists must first pass each other in front of your chest). Breathe out, stretch your right leg to right and turn your body to the left, keeping your left leg bent and your right leg straight. At the same time thrust hand forever in front of you and place your left hand on your right elbow. Breathe in, return to standing position. Repeat in opposite direction. Repeat this cycle 4 times.

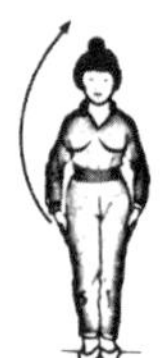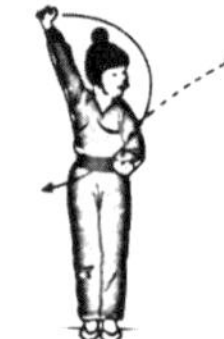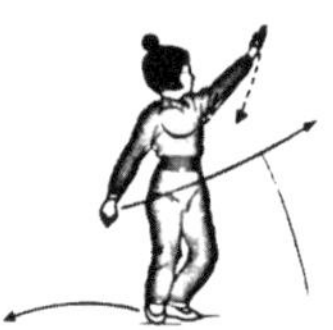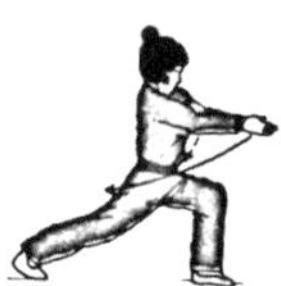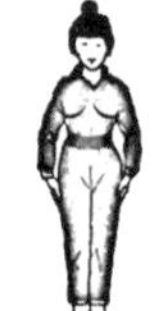

Breathe in, stand with your feet together, legs straight, arms slightly bent to your side, chest out and stomach in. Breathe out, keeping your knees together, come into a squatting position; while at the same time stretch your arms in front and shove your left fist into your right palm. Breathe in, stepping to your left while keeping your right leg straight, and bending you left leg, while at the same time spreading your arms to side with your palms facing up, keep your eyes on the left hand. Breathe out, turning to your right, while keeping your left leg straight, bend your right leg. At the same time place your left fist on your right knee, with palm facing out lift your right fist straight up above your head. Breathe in, return to standing position. Repeat in opposite direction. Repeat this cycle 4 times.

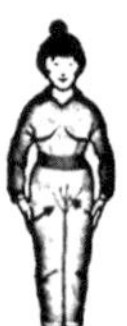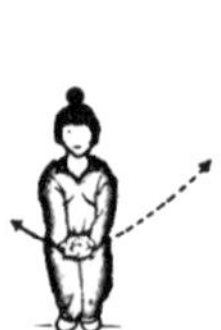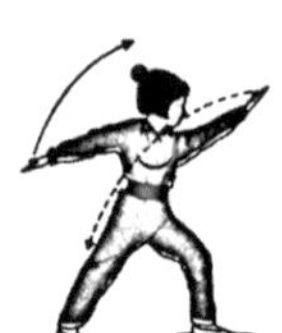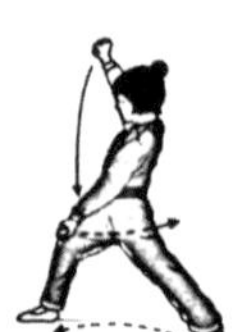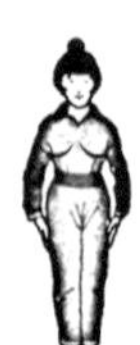

Breathe in, stand with your feet together, legs straight, arms slightly bent to your side, chest out and stomach in. Breathe out, stretching your right leg to your right, turn your body to the left and with your right leg straight, bend your left leg. At the same time, thrust your right hand forward in front of you, and keep your left hand at your waist, with your palm facing up. Breathe in, turning to your right and with your left leg straight, bend your right leg. At the same time pass your left hand above your right elbow and spread your arms to the side. With your palms facing forward. Breathe out, with your right leg still bent bring your left foot close to your right foot, and lift your heel off the ground, while at the same time raise your right arm, palm facing up, and stretch your left arm behind your back with your left wrist hooked upwards. Breathe in, come back to standing position. Repeat in the opposite direction. Repeat this cycle 4 times.

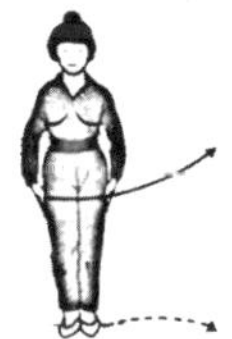 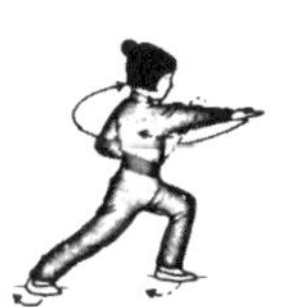 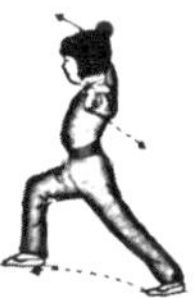 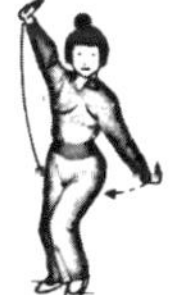 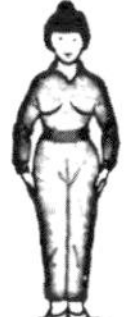

Breathe in, stand with your feet together, legs straight, arms slightly bent to your side, chest out and stomach in. Breathe out, step to the left, turning your body to the left and keeping your right leg straight, bend your left leg, while at the same time push your right fist forward in front of you, with your palm facing down, and hold your left fist at your waist, you're your palm facing

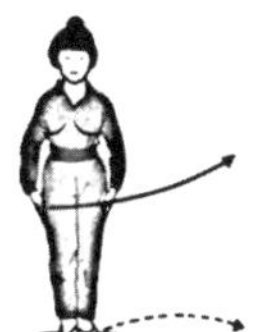 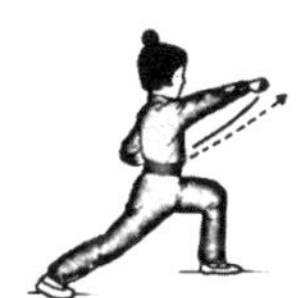 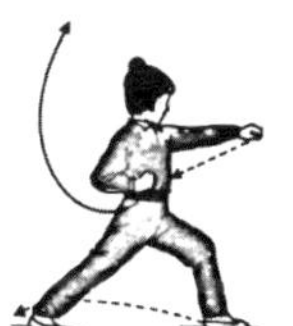 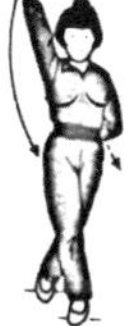 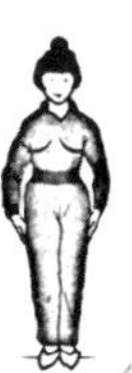

upward. Breathe in, pushing your left fist forward and bring your right fist to your waist. Breathe out, putting your weight on your right foot, draw your left foot behind you with only your toes touching the ground; while at the same time push your right fist down to the right of you and lift it up in a curve; resting your left fist behind you on your small of the back. Breathe in, come back into standing position. Repeat in the opposite direction. Repeat this cycle 4 times.

Breathe in, stand with your feet together, legs straight, arms slightly bent to your side, chest out and stomach in. Breathe out, step to your left, keeping your right leg straight, bend your left leg, while at the same time raise your arms to shoulder level and clap your hands. Breathe out, lower your hands to your waist and clench your fists, with palms facing up; while at the same time, keeping your legs straight, kick your right foot in the air in front of you. Breathe in, lower your right foot behind you and the right leg straight and with the left leg bent keeping your clenched fist to your waists and palms facing upward. Breathe out, push your fists forward in front of you with your palms facing each other. Breathe in, return to standing position. Repeat in the opposite direction. Repeat this cycle 4 times.

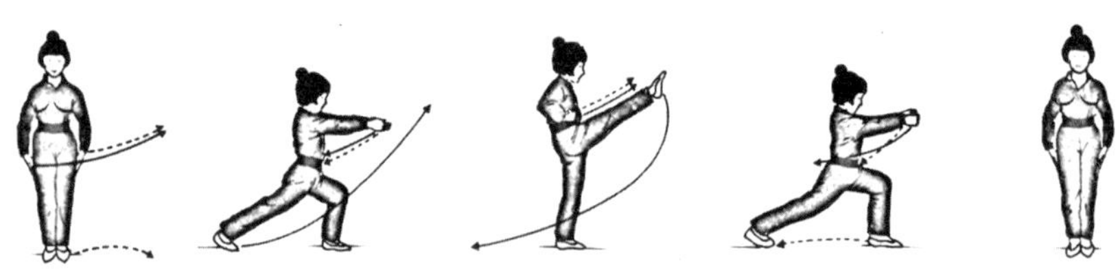

Office Movements – Section Two
Set One

Clenched Fists – Breathe in, standing with your feet shoulder-width apart, clench your fists and point your thumbs toward your thighs. Relax your shoulders and chest, looking straight ahead of you, with you mouth closed, and tongue touching your plate, concentrate on your lower abdominal area. Breathe out, tightening your clenched fists. Breathe in, and come back into standing position with your arms resting to your side Repeat this cycle 4 times.

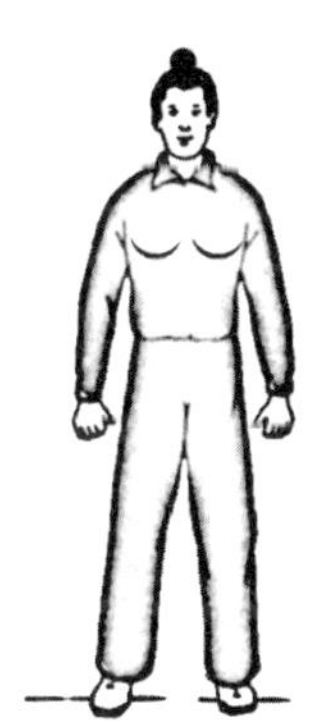

Hands Pressing Down – Breathe in, standing with your feet shoulder-width apart, arms hanging by your side, palms facing down and fingers pointing out away from your body, press down with your palms like you are pushing down on something. Breathe out; bend your finger upward so your whole body becomes tense. Breathe in, and come back into standing position with your arms resting to your side. Repeat this cycle 4 times.

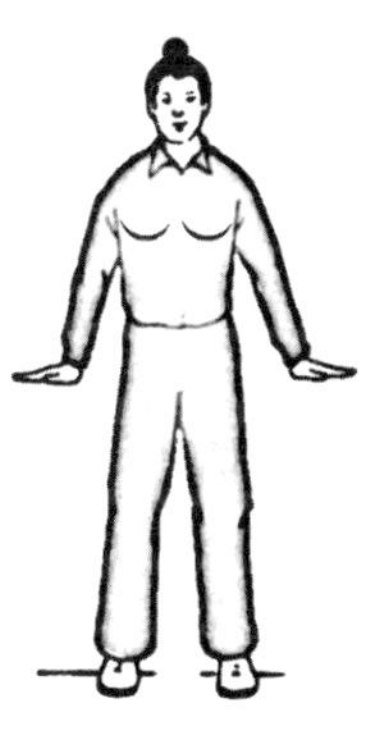

Palms Facing Up – Breathe in, standing with your feet shoulder-width apart. Stretch your arms to the side in a T – position with your palms facing up and tense your whole body. Breathe in, and come back into standing position with your arms resting to your side. Repeat this cycle 4 times.

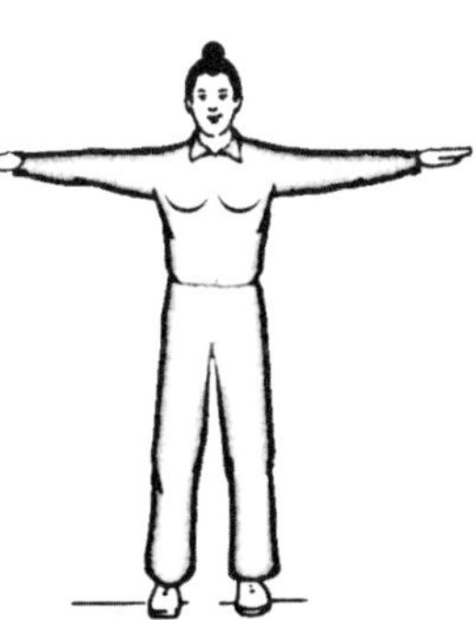

Palms Pressing Down – Breathe in, standing with your feet shoulder-width apart, Stretch your arms to the side in a T – position with your palms facing out and your hand is pointing upward. Breathe out. Pressing your palms outward tense your whole body. Breathe in, and come back into standing position. Repeat this cycle 4 times.

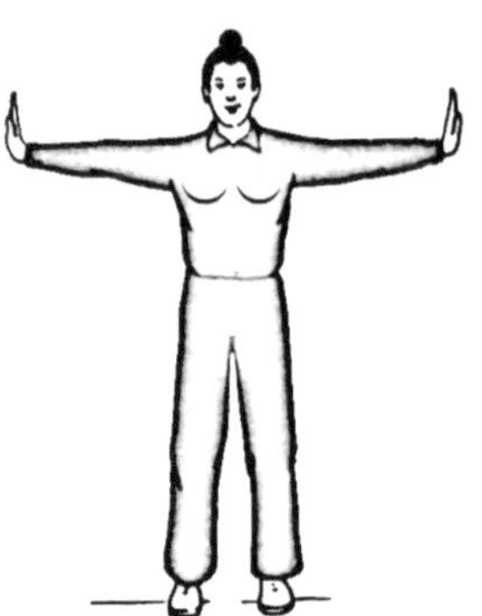

Palms Together and Apart – Breathe in, standing with your feet shoulder-width apart, bringing your palms together fingers pointing upward, with your palms close to your chest. Breathe out, bringing your palms apart pulling your thumbs along your chest until you reach the side of your chest. Breathe in, and come back into standing position with your arms resting to your side.. Repeat this cycle 4 times.

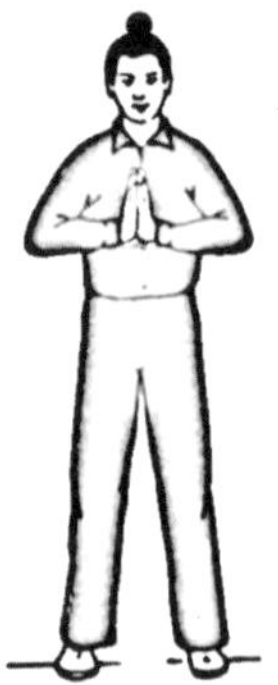

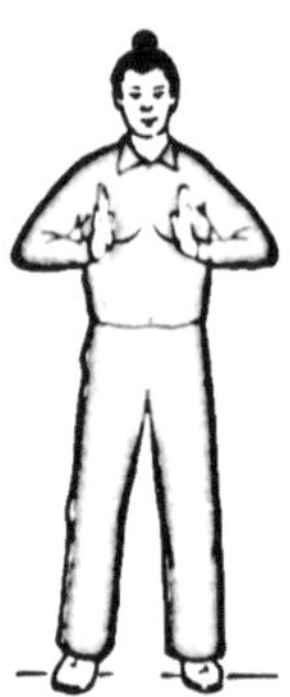

One Arm Up – Breathe in, standing with your feet shoulder-width apart, step to your left, bending your left leg and keeping your right leg straight and your upper body straight. Raise your left arm up with your left hand pointing upwards, palm facing outward, dropping your right arm hand pointing downward and palm facing inward. Tense your whole body as you pull your left hand up and your right hand down. Breathe out; turn your body to the right, bending your right leg, keeping your left leg straight and your upper body straight. Raise your right arm up with your right hand pointing upwards, palm facing outward, dropping your left arm, hand pointing downward and palm facing inward. Tense your whole body as you pull your right hand up and your left hand down. Breathe in, and come back into standing position with your arms resting to your side. Repeat this cycle 4 times.

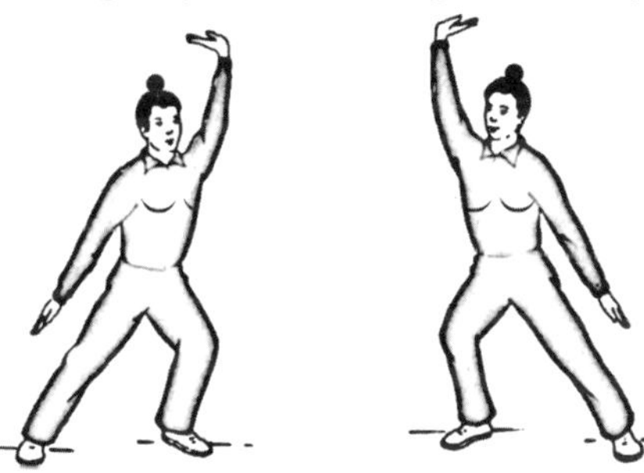

Sitting in a Chair – Breathe in, standing with your feet shoulder-width apart, stretch your arms in front of you with palms facing down, bending your knees until you are half way down. Imagine yourself sitting on a chair. Breathe out, pushing up from the sitting position arms stretch our out in front of you, palms facing down. Breathe in, and come back into a standing position with feet shoulder width apart, with your arms resting to your side.. Repeat this cycle 4 times.

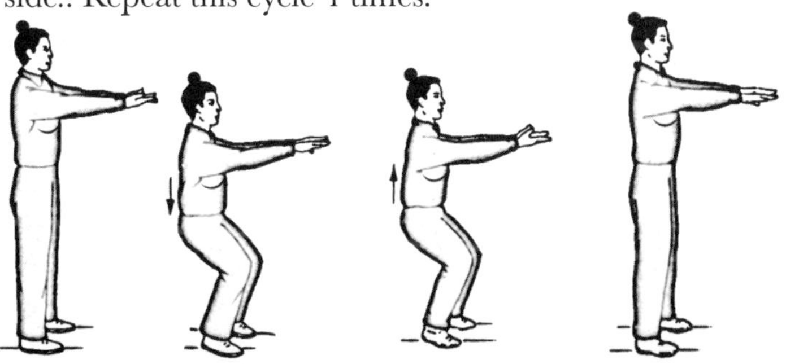

Sitting in a Chair II – Breathe in, standing with your feet shoulder-width apart, Place both arms behind your back holding your right fist with your left hand, bending your knees until you are half way down. Imagine yourself sitting on a chair. Breathe out, pushing up from the sitting position with arms still behind your back. Once legs are straight release your hands. Breathe in, and come back into a standing position with feet shoulder width apart, with your arms resting to your side. Repeat this cycle 4 times.

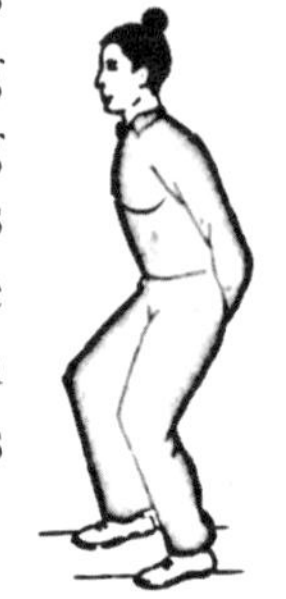

Bending Forward – Breathe in, standing with your feet shoulder-width apart, bend your upper body forward slowly, with your arms hanging loosely to your side, shoulders relaxed, palms facing your body, and fingers pointing downward. Remember as you bend down try to bend from the waist down and try not to curve your spine too much. Breathe out, pushing up and roll your upper torso upwards, hands hanging to your side, shoulders relaxed, head close to your chest, until your upper torso is straight again. Breathe in, and come back into a standing position with feet shoulder width apart, with your arms resting to your side.. Repeat this cycle 4 times.

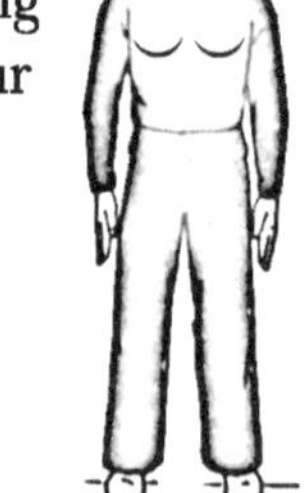

Side-backward Twist – Breathe in, standing with your feet shoulder-width apart, step to your left, bending your left leg, keeping your right leg straight, twist to your left , placing your left hand behind your back on the small of the back, palm facing out; curve your right arm over your head, palm facing down, a hand away from your face. Breathe out, bring your right arm back to your side, while you bring your left hand from your back and step back to center. Breathe in, come back into a standing position with feet shoulder width apart, with your arms resting to your side.. Repeat this cycle 4 times.

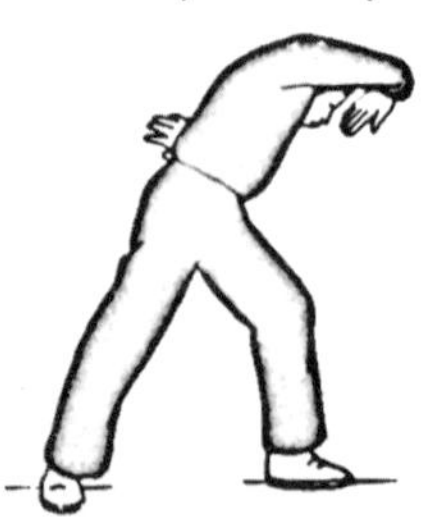

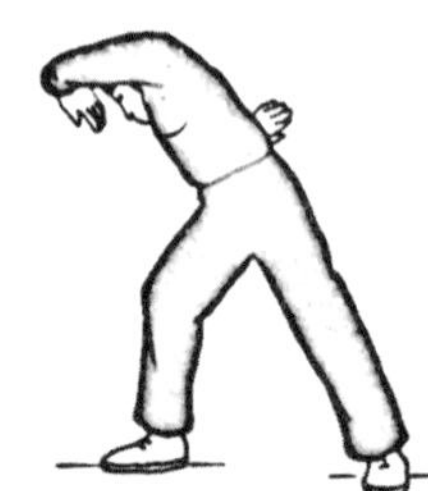

Set Two

Prayer Position – Breathe in, standing with your feet shoulder-width apart, bring your hands in prayer position, pressing your palms together. Breathe out, separating your palms about 2 inches (6cms). Breathe in; come back into standing position with your feet shoulder-width apart. Repeat this cycle 4 times.

Pushing Two Walls – Breathe in, standing with your feet shoulder-width apart, bring your hands in prayer position, pressing your palms together. Stretch your arms slowly out to the side with your palms facing out with your fingers pointing upward. Imagine you are pushing against two walls.. Breathe out; bring your hands back to prayer position. Breathe in; come back into standing position with your feet shoulder-width apart. Repeat this cycle 4 times.

Pushing to the Sky – Breathe in, standing with your feet shoulder-width apart, bring your hands in prayer position, pressing your palms together. Breathe out, raise your arms above your head with your elbows straight, palms facing upward, and fingers pointing to each other; stretch your whole body as if you want to touch the sky. Breathe in; bring your hands back to prayer position. Breathe out; come back into standing position with your feet shoulder-width apart. Repeat this cycle 4 times.

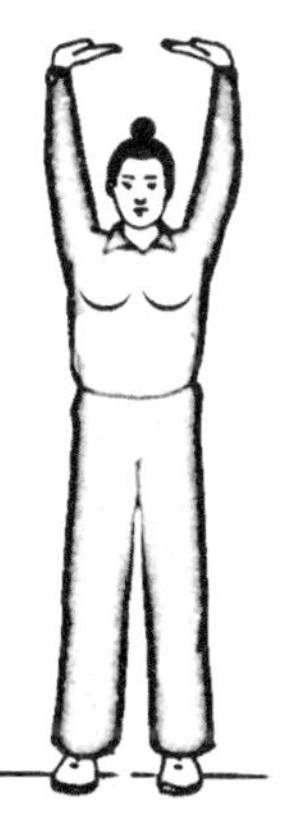

Pushing one Arm Up To the Sky – Breathe in, standing with your feet shoulder-width apart, bring your hands in prayer position, pressing your palms together. Raise your right hand above your head, palm down, keeping your eyes on your palm. Place your left hand behind you on the small of your back. Breathe out; bring your hands back to prayer position. Breathe in; come back into standing position with your feet shoulder-width apart. Repeat this cycle 4 times.

Pushing Against the Wall – Breathe in, standing with your feet together, bring your hands in prayer position, pressing your palms together. Stretch your arms out on front of you, palms upright away fro you with your fingers upward, with your head facing forward and looking at your hands. Imagine you are pushing against a wall. Breathe out; bring your hands back to prayer position. Breathe in; come back into standing position with your feet shoulder-width apart. Repeat this cycle 4 times.

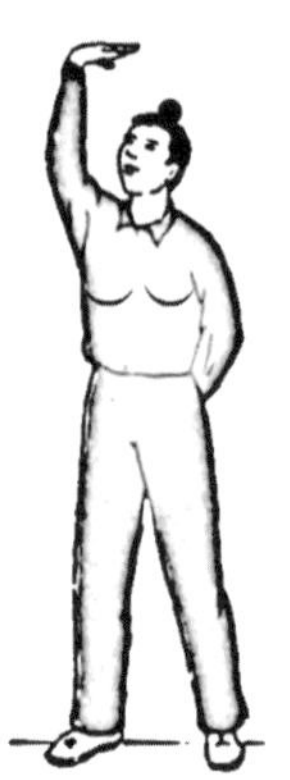

Leaning on the Wall – Breathe in, standing with your feet shoulder-width apart, bring your hands in prayer position, pressing your palms together, step to your right and turn your body to the right, bending your right leg and keeping your left leg straight. Raise your right arm bending your right elbow with your hand clenched into a fist, with your left arm bent and your left hand in a clench fist resting on your hip. Breathe out, coming back to center with your legs apart and your hands in prayer position. Breathe in, step to your left and turn your body to the left, bending your left leg and keeping your right leg straight. Raise your left arm bending your left elbow with your hand clenched into a fist, with your left arm bent and your left hand in a clench fist resting on your hip. Breathe out; bring your hands back to prayer position. Breathe in; come back into standing position with your feet shoulder-width apart. Repeat this cycle 4 times.

Arms Pulling Fingers Locked – Breathe in, standing with your feet shoulder-width apart, bring your hands in prayer position, pressing your palms together, place your left hand behind your back, with your palm facing out and your fingers reaching up as far as possible. Place your right hand over your shoulder and reach for the fingers of the left hand and pull the left fingers upward. Breathe out, come back into standing position with your feet apart shoulder width apart and your hands in prayer position.

Place your right hand behind your back, with your palm facing out and your fingers reaching up as far as possible. Place your left hand over your shoulder and reach for the fingers of the right hand and pull the right fingers upward. Breathe in; bring your hands back to prayer position. Breathe out; come back into standing position with your feet shoulder-width apart. Repeat this cycle 4 times.

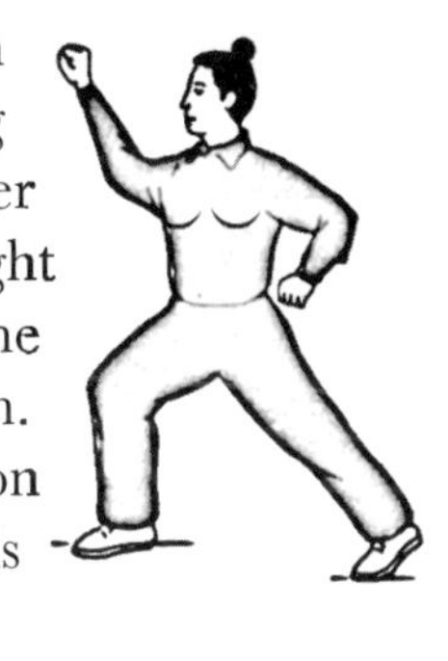

Sitting in Chair – Breathe in; come into standing position with your feet apart shoulder width apart and your hands in prayer position. Breathe out, step to the left and bend your knees to as if you were sitting in a chair, keeping your upper body straight, stretch your arms out to the side, palms facing upward. Breathe in and out, breathe in and out, and breathe in and out. Breathe in, and straighten back up into a standing position and into prayer position with feet shoulder width apart. Breathe out, step to the right and bend your knees to as if you were sitting in a chair, keeping your upper body straight, stretch your arms out to the side, palms facing down Breathe in and out, breathe in and out, and breathe in and out. Breathe in, and straighten up back into a standing position and into prayer position with feet shoulder width apart. Repeat this cycle 4 times.

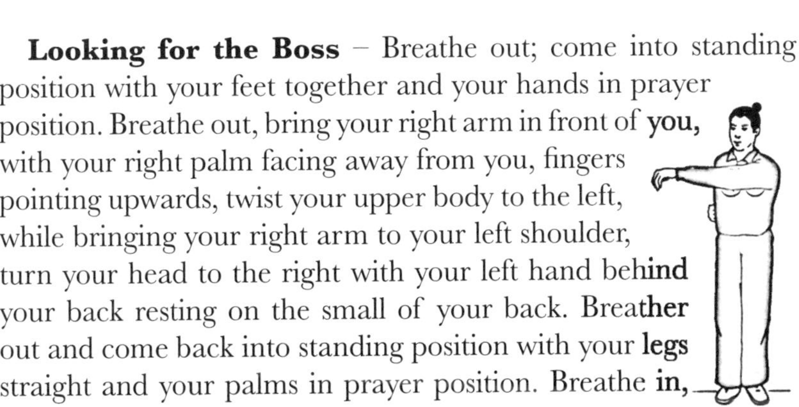

Looking for the Boss – Breathe out; come into standing position with your feet together and your hands in prayer position. Breathe out, bring your right arm in front of you, with your right palm facing away from you, fingers pointing upwards, twist your upper body to the left, while bringing your right arm to your left shoulder, turn your head to the right with your left hand behind your back resting on the small of your back. Breathe out and come back into standing position with your legs straight and your palms in prayer position. Breathe in, bring your left arm in front of you, with your left palm facing away from you, fingers pointing upwards, twist your upper body to the right, while bringing your left arm to your right shoulder, turn your head to the left with your right hand behind your back resting on the small of your back. Breathe out, come back into standing position with your hands in prayer. Repeat this cycle 4 times.

Touch the Floor – Breathe in; come into standing position with your feet apart shoulder-width apart and your hands in prayer position. Breathe out, step to the right and, with your left leg straight, bend your right knee. Bend down to your right, keeping your head up, touch the ground with both hands. Breathe in, straighten your arms and lift up your chest; bend your arms, twist your body to the left, bend your right elbow resting your right hand on your bent right knee, bend your left arm and place your left hand over your right hand on your right knee, while turning your head to the left. Breathe out; come back into standing position with your feet apart shoulder-width apart and your hands in prayer position. Breathe in, step to the left and, with your right leg straight, bend your left knee. Bend down to your left, keeping your head up, touch the ground with both hands. Breathe out, straighten your arms and lift up your chest; bend your arms, twist your body to the right, bend your left elbow resting your left hand on your bent left knee, bend your right arm and place your right hand over your left hand on your left knee, while turning your head to the right. Breathe in; come back into standing position with your feet apart shoulder-width apart and your hands in prayer position. Repeat this cycle 4 times.

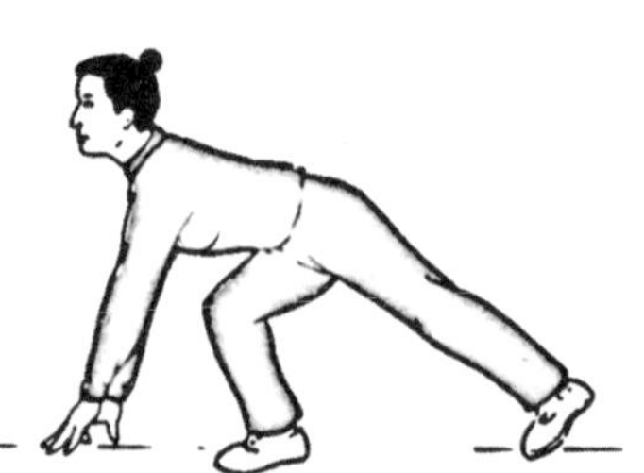
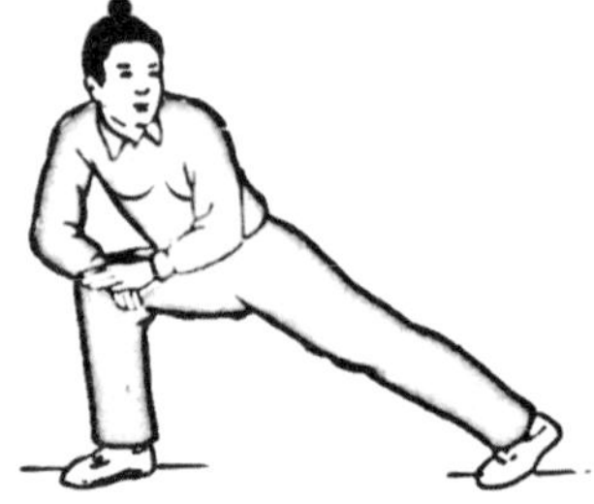

Head to Knee – Breathe in, come into standing position with your feet apart shoulder-width apart and your hands in prayer position. hold the back of head tightly with both your hands. Bending from your waist, keeping your back as straight as possible, bend your upper torso bringing your head to your knees. Breathe out; bring both your hands down to touch to your toes. Breathe in; stretch your hands out in front of you, stretching your upper torso out, lift both your hands above your head. Breathe in; come back into standing position with your feet apart shoulder-width apart and your hands in prayer position. Repeat this cycle 4 times.

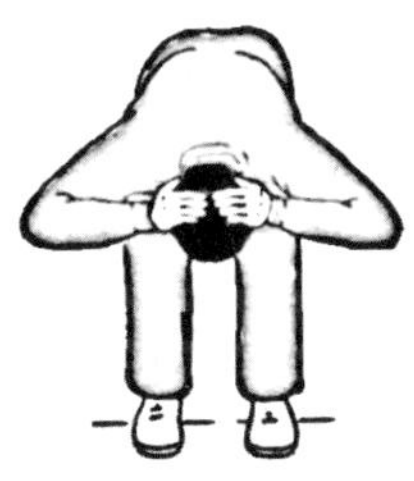

Set Three

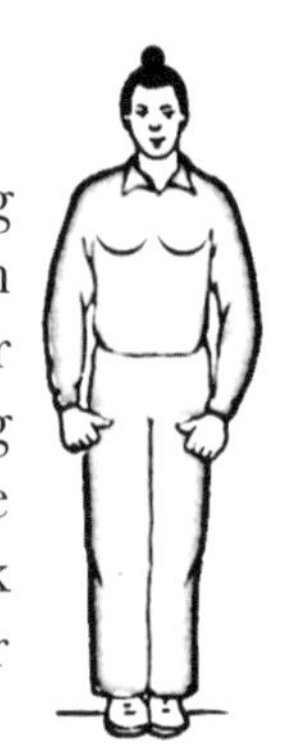

Thumb Lifting – Breathe in; come into standing position with your feet together with your hands in prayer position. Place your hands, in front of your thighs in a clenched fist position, with thumbs pointing at each other. Breathe out; tense your whole body while lifting your thumbs upward. - Breathe in; come back into standing position with your feet together and your hands in prayer position. Repeat this cycle 4 times.

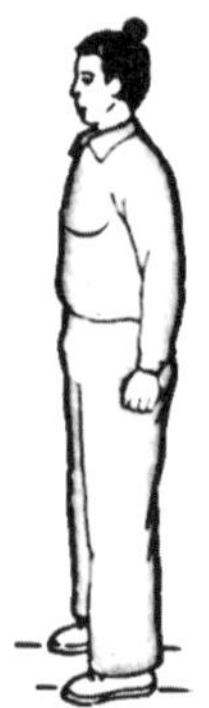

Thumb Holding -- Breathe in; come into standing position with your feet together with your hands in prayer position. Place your hands, in front of your thighs in a clenched fist position, with thumbs pointing at each other. Breathe out, bring thumbs into your clenched hands and tense your whole body. Breathe in; come back into standing position with your feet together and your hands in prayer position. Repeat this cycle 4 times.

Arms forward – Breathe in; come into standing position with your feet together with your hands in prayer position. Place your hands, in front of your body, with clenched fists, bending your thumbs into your hands and tense your whole body. Breathe in; come back into standing position with your feet together and your hands in prayer position. Repeat this cycle 4 times.

Arms Upward – Breathe in; come into standing position with your feet apart and your hands in prayer position. Raise your arms slowly above your head, with your hands in clenched fists, bending your thumbs into hands, fists facing each other, while stretching your arms behind your head and tense your whole body. Breathe in; come back into standing position with your feet together and your hands in prayer position. Repeat this cycle 4 times.

Clench Hands to Ears – Breathe in; come into standing position with your feet apart with your heels touching and your hands in prayer position. Raise your arms slowly to your ears, with your hands in clenched fists, bending your thumbs into hands, fists facing your ears, and tense your whole body. Breathe in; come back into standing position with your feet together and your hands in prayer position. Repeat this cycle 4 times.

Toe Lifting – Breathe in; come into standing position with your feet apart, with your heels touching and your hands in prayer position. Raise your arms slowly to your shoulders, with your hands in clenched fists, bending your thumbs into hands, stretch your arms away from your body in a T position, while you life your toes off the ground, tense your whole body. Breathe in; come back into standing position with your feet together and your hands in prayer position. Repeat this cycle 4 times.

Clench Hands to Nose – Breathe in; come into standing position with your feet apart with your heels touching and your hands in prayer position. Raise your arms slowly bending your elbows 45 degrees toward your nose, hands in clenched fists, bending your thumbs into hands, fists facing your nose, and tense your whole body. Breathe in; come back into standing position with your feet together and your hands in prayer position. Repeat this cycle 4 times.

Clench Upright – Breathe in; come into standing position with your feet apart, with your heels touching and your hands in prayer position. Raise your arms slowly to your shoulders, with your hands in clenched fists, bending your thumbs into hands, stretch your arms away from your body in a T position, bend your arms to 90 degrees, while you life your toes off the ground, tense your whole body. Breathe in; come back into standing position with your feet together and your hands in prayer position. Repeat this cycle 4 times.

Clench Fists to Navel – Breathe in; come into standing position with your feet apart, with your heels touching and your hands in prayer position. Raise your arms slowly to your shoulders, with your hands in clenched fists, bending your thumbs into hands, stretch your arms away from your body in a T position, bend your arms to 90 degrees, while you life your toes off the ground, tense your whole body. Breathe in; come back into standing position with your feet together and your hands in prayer position. Repeat this cycle 4 times.

Clench Fists by Chest – Breathe in; come into standing position with your feet apart, with your heels touching and your hands in prayer position. Raise your arms slowly to your shoulders, with your hands in clenched fists, bending your thumbs into hands, stretch your arms away from your body in a T position, bend your arms to 90 degrees, while you life your toes off the ground, tense your whole body. Breathe in; come back into standing position with your feet together and your hands in prayer position. Repeat this cycle 4 times.

Fifteen Minute Movements
Section Three

Head – Breathe in; come into a standing position with your feet apart, arms bent with your hands resting on your hips, drop your head toward your chest. Breathe out, bring your head back to center and stretch your head back as far as possible and bring your head back to center. Breathe in, turn your head to the right, with your chin as close to your right shoulder, and bring your head back to center. Breathe out; turn your head to the left with your chin as close to your left shoulder. Come back to center. Breathe in, rotating your head from left to right, chin to your chest, left ear to your shoulder, head back as possible, right ear to your shoulder, chin to your chest, and back to center. Remember to keep your upper torso facing forward. Your head should be the only thing that is motion. Breathe out, rotating your head to the right, chin to your chest, right ear to your shoulder, head back as possible, left ear to your shoulder, chin to your chest, and back to center. Repeat this cycle 4 times.

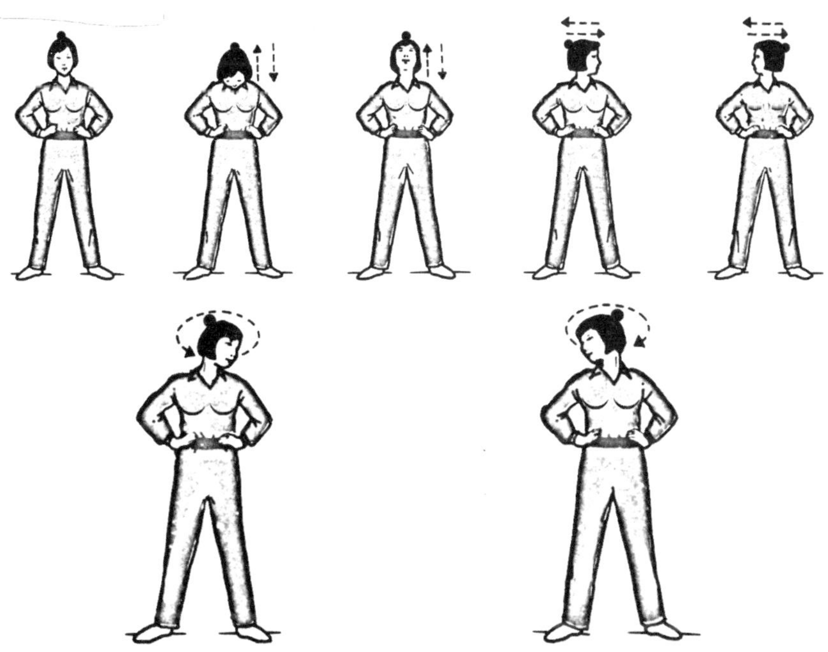

Arms – Breathe in; come into a standing position with your feet together arms bent with your hands resting on your hips, bring your hands in front of you and interlock them, stretch your arms in front of you pushing down with your palms open. Breathe out; with your fingers still interlocked and elbows bent, bring your hands to your chest. Stretch your arms straight out with backs of your hands facing your body. Bend your elbows and bring your hands back to chest. Breathe in, stretching your arms straight out again with backs of your hands facing your body and bend your elbows and bring your hands back to chest. Breathe out; come back to the standing position with your feet apart, arms straight with your hands resting by your side. Repeat this cycle 4 times.

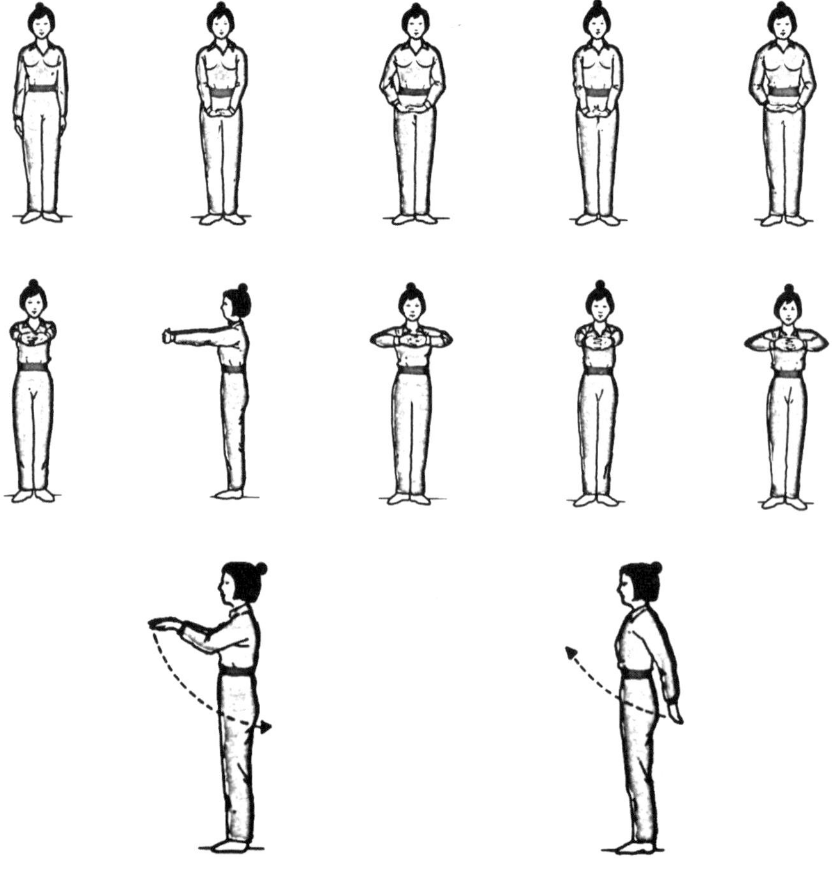

Chest – Breathe in; come into a standing position with your feet together, arms straight with your hands resting by your sides. Breathe out; step forward with your left leg and shift your weight to the left foot. With your right leg is behind lift your right heel off the ground and bring your hands up to your chest pointing at each other, with your palms facing down. Breathe in; keeping your up and chest out, move your arms down and up like you want to fly. Remember to keep your chest out as far possible and when lifting arms up and down, keep your arms straight Repeat this cycle 4 times.

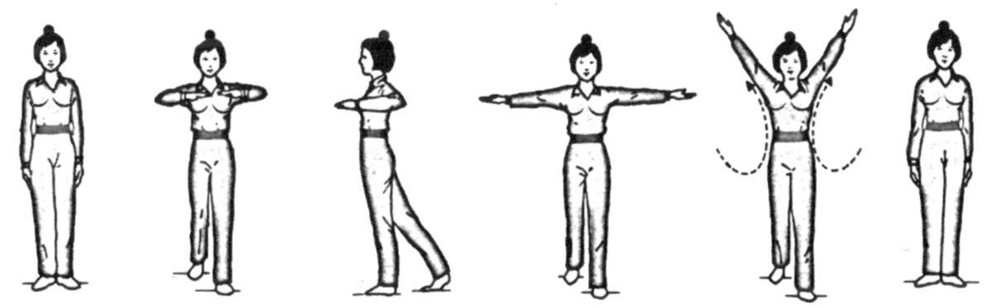

Legs – Breathe in; come into a standing position with your feet together, arms straight with your hands resting by your sides. Breathe out, put your hands on your hips with your elbows bent, lift your left leg with your knee bent and kick forward. Breathe in, lower your left leg. Breathe out, lift your right leg with your knee bent and kick forward. Breathe in, lower the right leg. Breathe out; come back into a standing position and bring your arms to your side. Repeat this cycle 4 times.

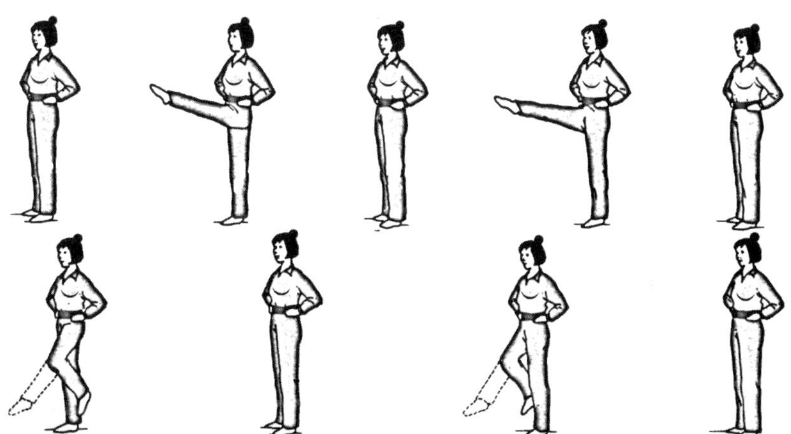

Sides – Breathe in; come into a standing position with your feet together, arms straight with your hands resting by your sides. Breathe out; step to your left and stretch your arms in T-position palms facing down. Breathe in, stretch your right arm high above head, bending your body to the left. Put your left arm down behind you back and lift your left foot up so that only the toes are touching. Breathe in; come back into a standing position with your feet together, arms straight with your hands resting by your sides. Breathe out; step to your right and stretch your arms in T-position palms facing down. Breathe in, stretch your left arm high above head, bending your body to the right. Put your right arm down behind you back and your right foot up so that only the toes are touching. Breathe out; come back into a standing position and bring your arms to your side. Repeat this cycle 4 times.

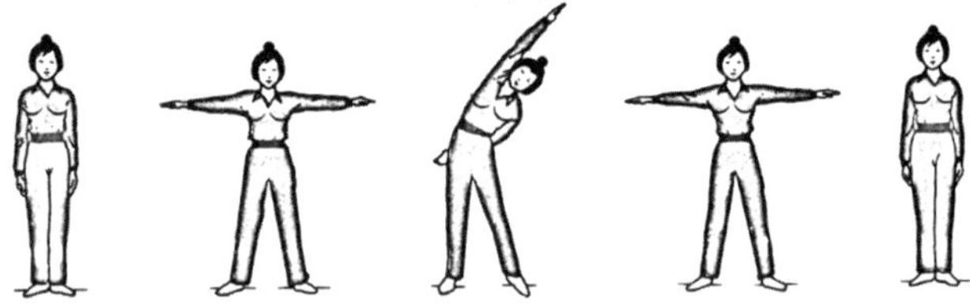

Body –Twisting Breathe in; come into a standing position with your feet together, arms straight with your hands resting by your sides. Breathe out, stretch your arms out in front of your body, and clench your fists, with your palms facing down. Breathe in; step to your left twisting your body to the left together with your left arm, palm facing forward while at the same time bend your right arms, palm facing down close to your chest. Breathe out; bring your arms stretch out in front of your body. Breathe in, step to your right twisting your body to the right together with your right arm, palm facing forward while at the same time bend your left arms, palm facing down close to your chest. Breathe out; bring your arms stretch out in front of your body. Breathe in, come back to standing position with your feet together, arms straight with your hands resting by your sides. Repeat this cycle 4 times.

The Whole Body – Breathe in; come into a standing position with your feet together, arms straight with your hands resting by your sides. Breathe out; raise both your arms, palms facing out with your fingers pointing upward. Keeping your head high and your chest out bend your upper body back with your stretched arms behind your head and return your arms along side your head. Keeping arms straight, bend your upper body again keeping your head looking forward stretch your arms behind your head and return your arms along side your head. Breathe in; with straight knees, bend your upper torso with your arms stretched out in front of you, bend forward from your waist and touch the ground. Bend your knees if you can't touch the ground with straight legs. Breathe out; stretching your arms in front of you raise your upper body slightly and bend your knees and come into a crouching position placing both hands on your knees. Breathe in; straighten your legs keeping your body bent forward and touch your knees. Breathe out, and come into a crouching position again with your hands resting on your knees. Breathe in, stretching your arms in front of you bend down again and touch the floor. Breathe out, stretching your arms out in front of you palms facing down and fingers pointing outward, raise your body upward arms coming to you're the side of your head. Breathe in; come back into a standing position with your feet together, arms straight with your hands resting by your sides. Repeat this cycle 4 times.

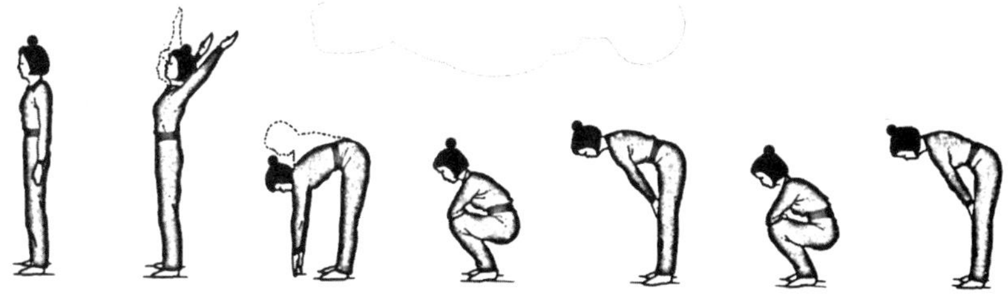

Limbering – Breathe in; come into a standing position with your feet together, arms straight with your hands resting by your sides. Breathe out; stretch arms to the side in T-position, palms down, lift your left knee. Breathe in; come back in to standing position and cross your arms in front of your body. Breathe out; stretch arms to the side in T-position, palms down, lift your right knee. Breathe in; come back in to standing position and cross your arms in front of your body. Breathe out; stretch arms to the side in T-position, palms down, swing you're your left leg sideways. . Breathe in; come back in to standing position and cross your arms in front of your body. Breathe out; stretch arms to the side in T-position, palms down, swing your right leg sideways. Breathe in; come back in to standing position and cross your arms in front of your body. Breathe out; come back into a standing position with your feet together, arms straight with your hands resting by your sides. Repeat this cycle 4 times.

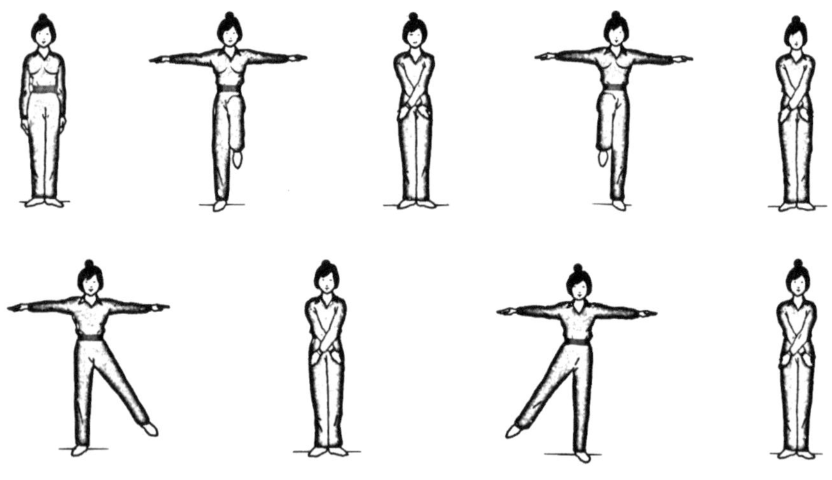

Neijia Inner Body Workouts

The internal body workouts, which emphasize slow movements and tranquility of mind, have a completely different emphasis to the external forms of exercise. The most popular of all internal exercises is Tai shadow boxing, known in China as Tapiquan. This is included here as well as Taiji swordplay and the Taiji duet.

The underlying principle of the internal exercises is the idea that action follows thought. An example of this is in the starting position, where the slow raising of arms occurs only after the thought of raising arms has occurred. All internal exercise are controlled by such consciousness and one must therefore be quiet and calm before beginning each exercise and then apply one's total concentration.

Relaxation is all-important. Muscles and joints should be relaxed to such a degree that all rigidity disappears. The torso should be kept upright with arms held in a rounded manner and legs bent or curved as required. Special attention must be paid to balance as one moves from one position to another and natural breathing is essential. The basic rule of 'up, inhale; down, exhale' naturally coordinates breathing with action. In the starting position, for example, the raising of the arms causes you to breathe in and the lowering of the arms to breathe out.

There are several distinguishing features of the internal forms of exercise. Lightness and suppleness characterize them all. Taiiquan should be done slowly and smoothly as the movements are in accord with the natural motions of the human body. After exercising one should feel relaxed and refreshed rather than exerted, and it is therefore especially suitable for the elderly, the infirm and sufferers of chronic diseases.

Continuity is important. Taijiquan from beginning to end should be a smooth, uninterrupted flow of movement. Movements of arms and hands in curves and arcs should follow the natural curves of your joints. This ensures an even exertion of each part of the body.

Finally, Taiiquan requires a close coordination of tht upper and lower parts of the body. Taijiquan also calls for harmony between inner and outer body movements and you must be aware of your breathing. Each movement involves the whole body, with the waist and back initiating the movement of your limbs. Such well-coordinated movements automatically eliminate any rigidity and disjointedness.

Pay special attention to certain parts of the body while doing these exercises. Move your head naturally with your torso, keep your chin in and mouth closed with your tongue resting gently behind your upper teeth, and breathe through your nose. Eyes should follow the hand that is in front and your neck should be neither too stiff nor too relaxed. Your chest should be pulled in and your shoulder should be kept low.

Gravity acts through your legs giving you firm contact with the ground, as can be seen by the constant shifting of weight from one leg to the other. Knee joints should be relaxed throughout, and even when told to keep legs straight the knee joints should never be locked. When advancing always touch the ground with your heel first and when retreating put your toe down first. The sinking of shoulders and lowering of elbows is especially important as, when these two joints are relaxed, arms and wrists become naturally curved and fingers naturally spread.

Shadow Boxing

Section 1 – Preparation

Stand to attention. Step to left so that feet are shoulder-width apart, relax arms and hold them by side. Keep head and neck up, pull abdomen in and look straight ahead. 2. Lower shoulders and slowly raise arms to shoulder level, palms down. 3. Lower elbows and wrists so that hands are upright. 4. Keep torso straight, bend knees and press hands down lightly, lower elbows toward knees.

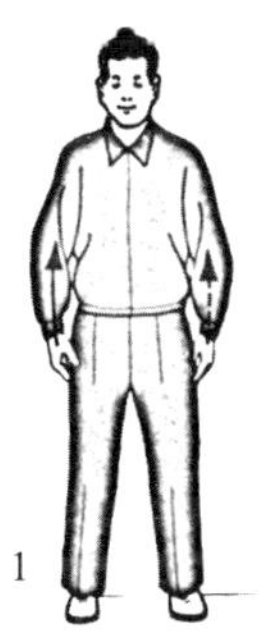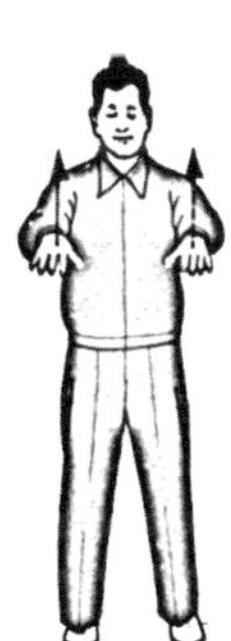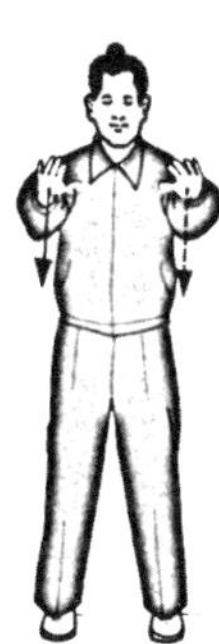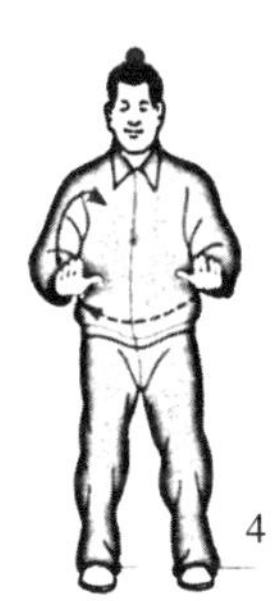

Parting of Wild Horse Mane

Turn torso slightly to right and put weight on right leg; at same time lift right hand, palm down, to chest level, and move left hand to right, palm up, and position hands as though holding a ball. 2. Move left foot, with heel raised, to right and keep eyes on right hand. 3. Turn torso slightly to left and step to left with left and right leg straight, bend left knee. 4-5. At same time move left hand up to eye level, palm up, elbow slightly bent, and right hand down to waist level, palm down, elbow slightly bent; keep eyes on left hand. 6. Slowly move torso back, shift weight to right leg and lift left toes off ground7. Move torso forward and to left, shifting weight to left leg, at same time draw left hand back toward chest, palm down, move right palm up and position hands as though holding a ball. 8. Bring right foot next to left foot, lift right heel off ground and keep eyes on left hand. 9-10. Move right foot forward to right and keeping left leg straight, bend right knee and repeat steps 4-5, but in opposite direction. 11-15. Repeat steps 1-5.

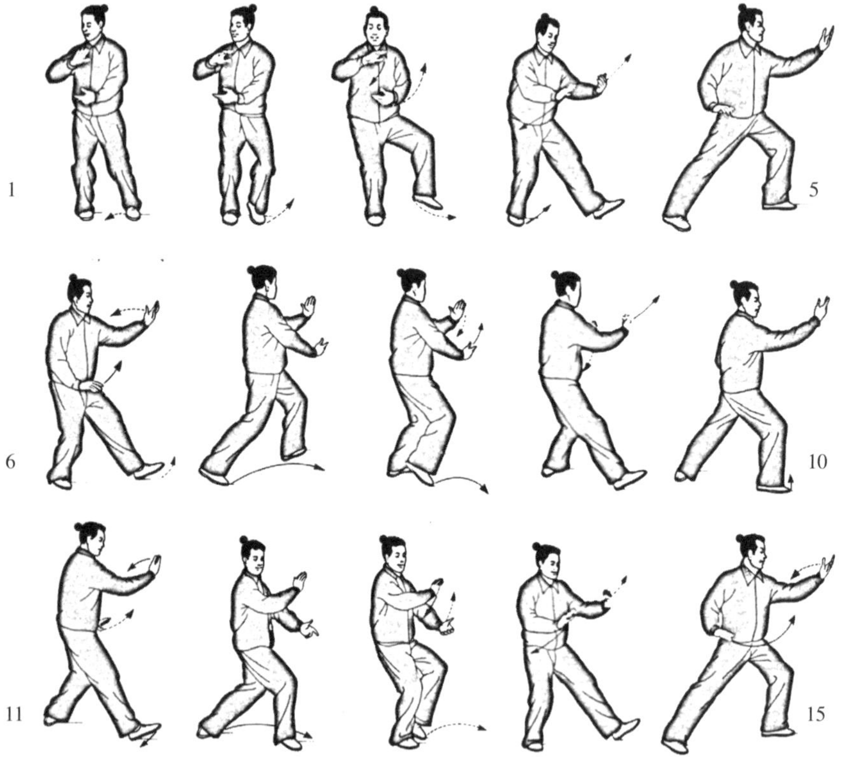

White Crane Flaps Its Wings

Turn torso slightly to left, lower left hand, palm down, and move right hand forward in a curse, palm up, and position hands as though holding a ball, keep eyes on left hand. 2. Move right foot half a step forward and shift weight back to right leg, at same time raise right hand to eye level, press down with left hand and turn torso to right. Move left foot forward, lift heel off ground and turn torso slightly to left; raise right hand to level of forehead, drop left hand, palm down, by left hip and look ahead.

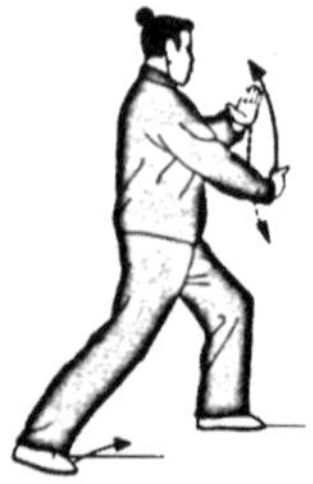

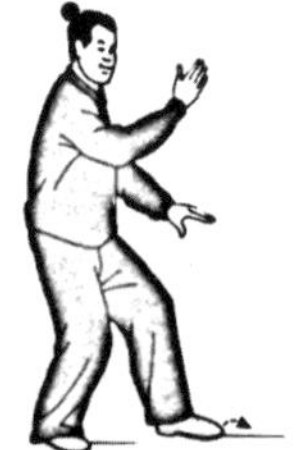

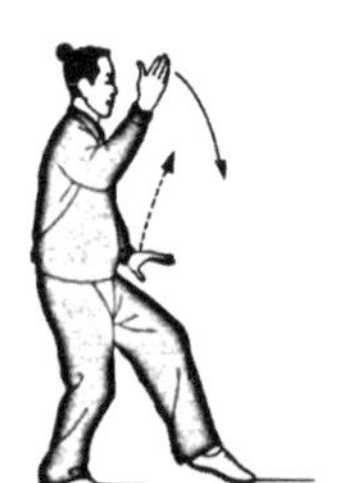

Section 2 – Brushing the Knee

1-3. Turn torso slightly to left and then to right, lower right hand and pass it along right hip before raising it in a curve to eye level, at same time move left hand up, then down in a curve to front of chest; at same time point toes of left foot toward ground and keep eyes on right hand. 4-5. Turn torso to left, step to left with left foot and keeping right leg straight, bend left leg; at same time as turning torso push right hand forward at nose level, brush left hand across left knee and hold it by left hip, palm down; keep eyes on fingers of right hand. 6-7. Bend right knee slowly, shift weight onto right leg and lift toes of left foot off ground. Turn torso to left and shift weight to left leg. 8. Bring right foot next to left foot and point toes of right foot toward ground, at same time turn left palm up and move it out to left. Follow turning of torso with right hand and bring it to right side of chest, palm down; keep eyes on left hand. 9-10. Repeat steps 4-5, but in opposite direction. 11-13. Repeat steps 6-8, but in opposite direction. 14-15. Repeat steps 4-5.

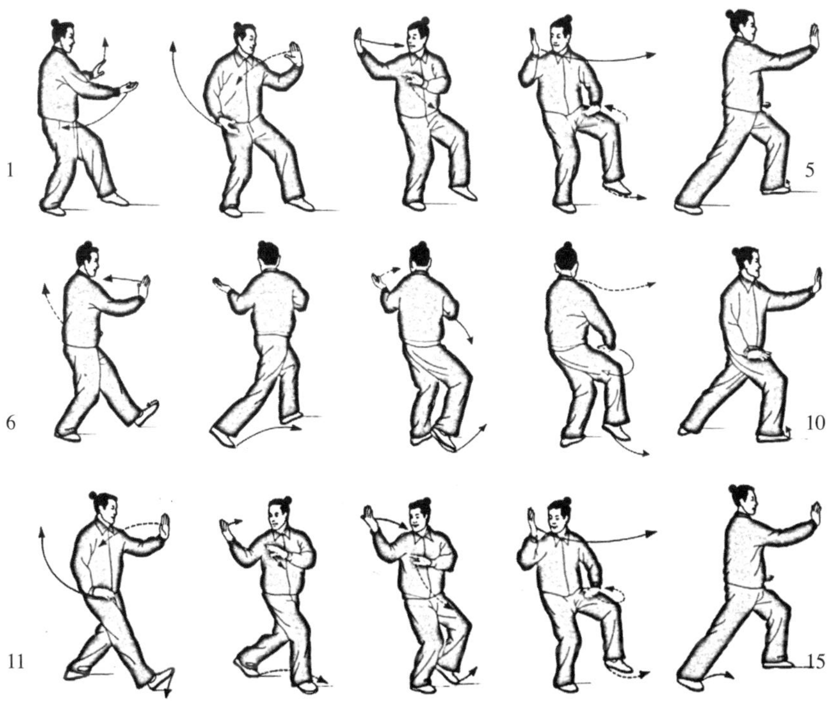

75

Curving Back Arms to Left and Right

1-2 Turn torso to right and draw right hand back and up in a curve with palm up and arm slightly bent. At same time turn left palm up, keep eyes to right as you turn torso and then turn to look at left hand. 3-4. Bend right elbow, push right hand forward, palm facing front; bend left elbow and draw left hand back to waist, palm up. At same time lift left foot and take one step back, shift weight onto left leg, keeping eyes on right hand. 5. Turn torso slightly to left and raise left hand in a backward curse, palm up; at same time turn right palm up, follow torso with eyes to left first and then turn to look at right hand. 6-8. Repeat steps 3-5, but in opposite direction9-10. Repeat steps 3-4. Repeat step 5. 12-13. Repeat steps 3-4, but in opposite direction.

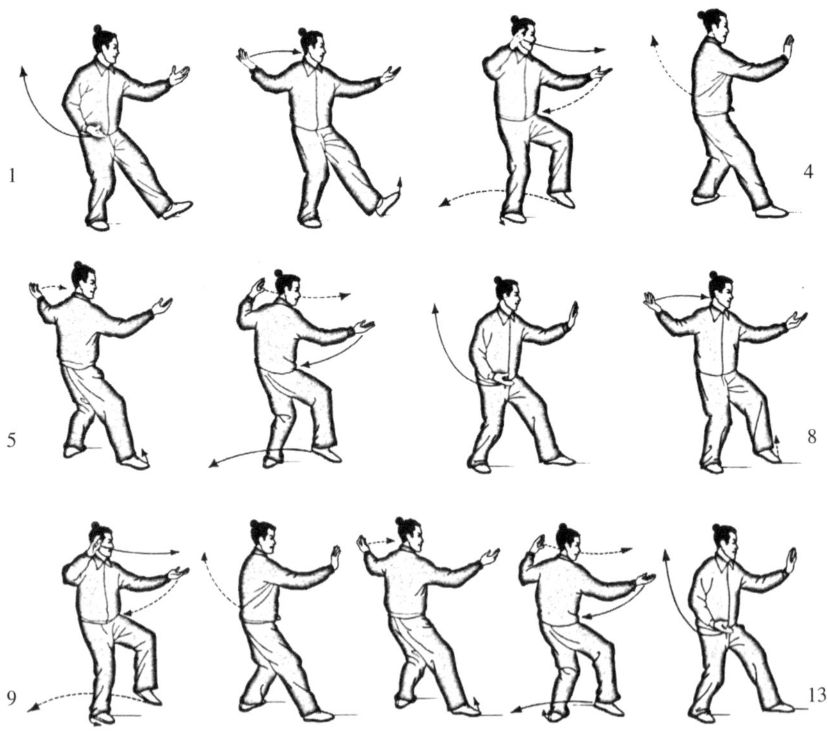

Strumming the Lute

1-3. Take half a step forward with right foot and lower torso, shifting weight onto right leg. Turn torso 90 degrees to right, lift left leg, move it forward and put it down with its toes off ground and knee slightly bent; at same time bring left hand up and forward to nose level, palm facing right, arm slightly bent, and draw right hand back to face inside of left elbow, palm facing left and keep eyes on left and thumb.

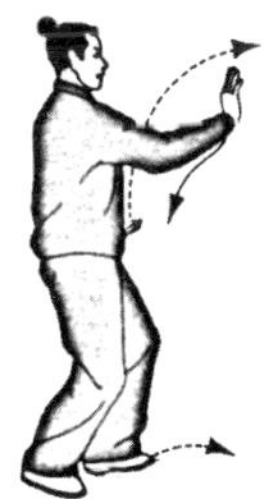 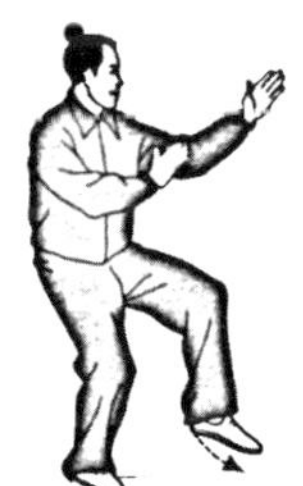 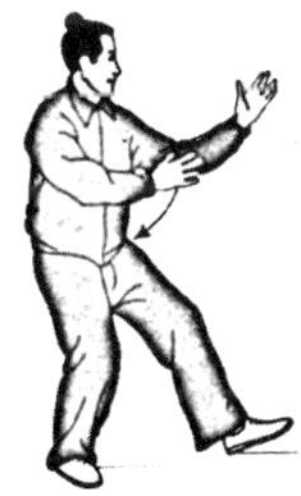

Section 3 – Grasping the Bird's Tail to the Left

Turn torso slightly to right and draw right hand back and up In a curve. Relax left hand, palm down, and keep eyes on it. 2-3. continue to turn torso to right, bring left hand down in a curse and hold it at rib cage, palm down, bring right arm in front of chest, palm down and position hands as though holding a ball. At same time put weight on right leg, draw left foot in, toes pointing toward ground, and keep eyes on right hand. 4-5. Turn torso slightly to left, step forward with left foot and keeping right leg straight, bend left knee, at same time move left forearm forward, palm facing body, and draw right hand back to hip, palm down. Keep eyes looking at left hand? 6-7. Turn left palm down and bring right palm up, turn to right and at same time move hands to right in a curve. Hold right hand at shoulder level, palm up, and bend left arm in front of body, palm facing chest. Shift weight onto right leg and keep eye on right hand. 8-9. Turn torso slightly to left, bend right elbow and bring right hand toward left wrist, palms facing each other. Look at left wrist and keeping right leg straight, bend left leg and put weight on left leg. 10-12. Turn left palm down and bring right hand over left wrist. Separate hands and hold them shoulder-width apart, palms down; at same time bend right knee, lower torso and shift weight onto right leg with toes of left foot lifted off ground. Lower elbows, bring hands back to abdomen, and look ahead. 13. Shift weight forward slowly keep right leg straight, bend left knee, push hands forward and look straight ahead.

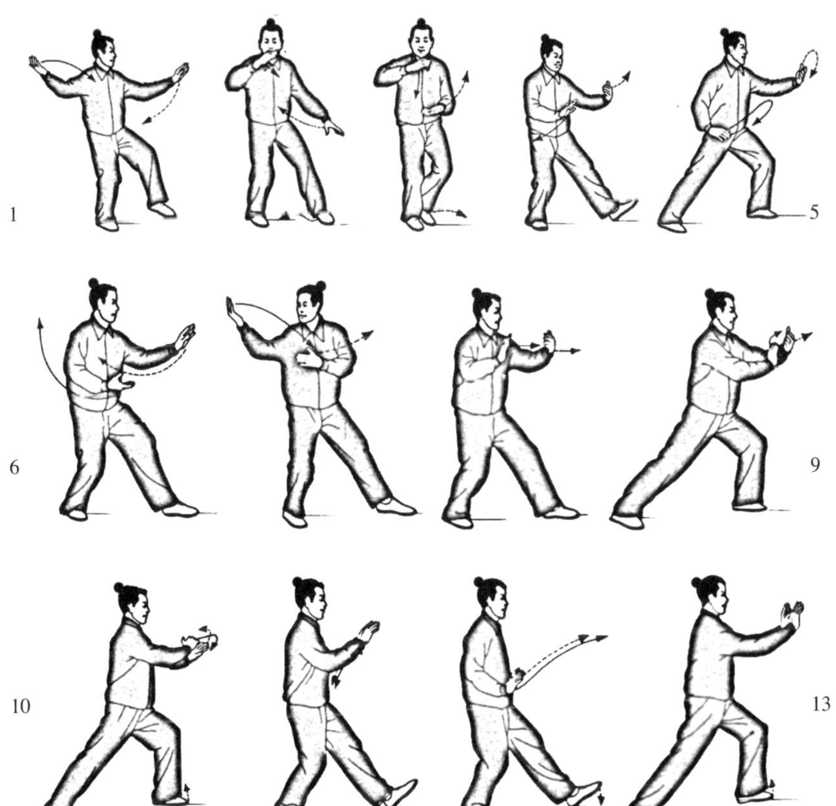

1
5
6
9
10
13

Grasping the Bird's Tail to the Right

1. Lower torso, turn to right, bring right foot with you and shift weight to right leg; lift left toes off ground and turn them in. 2. Bring right hand behind back in a curve, follow movement with eyes. 3-4. Shift weight onto left leg, bring right hand down in a curve, hold it in front of left ribs, hold left hand in front of chest, palm down, and position hands as though holding a ball; at same time draw right foot in with toes pointing to ground and keep eyes on left hand. 5-6.Repeat steps 4-5 of Grasping the bird's tail to the left, but in opposite direction. 7-10. Repeat steps 6-9 of grasping the bird's tail to the left, but in opposite direction. 11-14. Repeat steps 10-13 of grasping the bird's tail to the left, but in opposite direction.

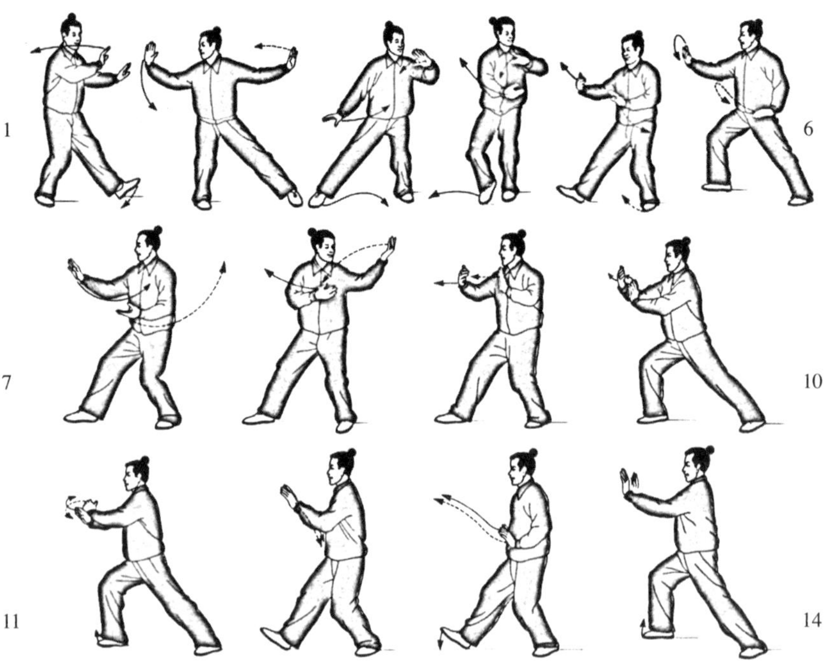

Section 4 – Single Whip

1. Lower torso, shift weight onto left leg and lift toes of right foot off ground and turn them in. 2. Turn torso to left, hold left hand at shoulder level, palm facing left, and right hand by left ribs, palm up; keep eyes on left hand. 3-4. Shift weight slowly to right leg while turning torso to right and drawing left foot in with only toes touching ground; At same time move right hand up in a curve to right at shoulder level, close fingers round thumb loosely and hang hand down from wrist joint. Pass left hand in front of abdomen to front of right shoulder. Keep eyes on left palm. 5-6. Turn torso to left, step forward with left foot and keeping left leg straight, bend right leg and shift weight onto left leg. At same time push left palm out, arm slightly bent, and keep eyes on left hand.

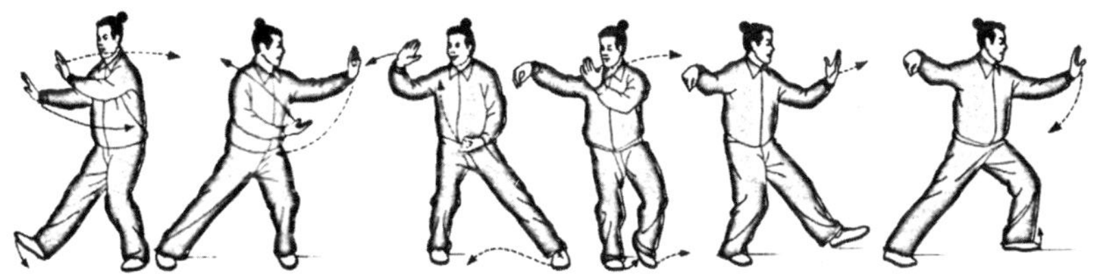

Waving the Hands in the Air

Return weight to right leg and gradually turn torso to right with left toes raised and turning in. 2-3. Pass left hand in front of abdomen, move it up in a curse and hold it in front of right shoulder, at same time unhook right hand and turn palm up to face out, keeping eyes on left palm. 4-6. Turn torso slowly to left, shift weight to left leg and draw right foot in so that it is parallel with the left foot, at same time move left hand in front of face to left, palm down in a curse and up to front of left shoulder, with eyes on right palm. 7-8. Turn torso to right and keeping weight on right leg, stretch left leg over lo left, at same time wave right hand to right, palm facing out, and move left hand down in a curve and up to front of right shoulder, keeping eyes on front of left shoulder. 9-11. Repeat steps 4-6. 12-13. Repeat steps 7-8. 14-16. Repeat steps 4-6.

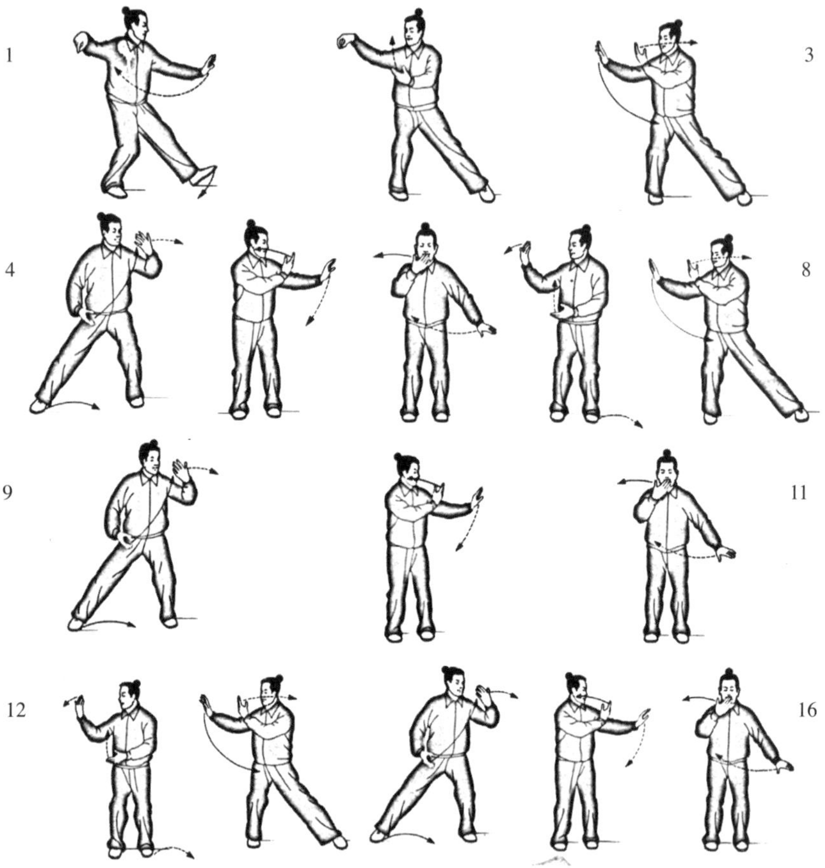

Single Whip – 1-2. Turn torso to right and follow movement with right hand; at same time pass left hand in front of abdomen and move it up in a curve to front of right shoulder, keeping eyes on left palm. Close fingers of right hand round thumb and hang hand from wrist joint, Shift weight to right leg and lift left heel so that toes remain touching ground. 3-4. Turn torso gradually to left, keep left hand at eye level, step to left with left foot and keeping left leg straight, bend right knee. Shift weight onto left leg and while continuing to turn torso to left, turn left palm to push outward, formatting a "Single whip" position.

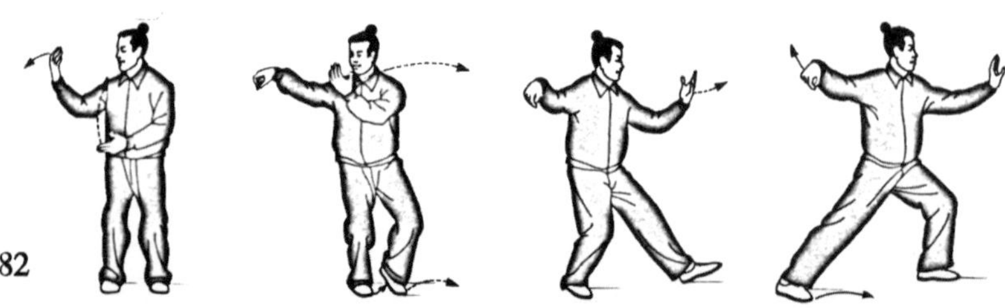

Section Five – Patting the Horse

Take half a step forward with right foot and gradually shift weight back to right leg. Open right hand and turn both palms up, elbows slightly bent; at same time lift left heel off ground and turn torso slightly to right. 2. Turn torso slightly to left, bring right hand past right ear and push forward, keeping fingers at eye level, at same time draw left hand back to waist, palm up, and step forward with left foot, heel raised off ground, keeping eyes on right hand.

Kicking With the Right Heel

1. Cross wrists by passing left hand, palm up, over right hand. 2-3. Uncross hands in a downward motion, palms down, and at same time raise left leg and step out to left. Keep right leg straight, bend left leg and shift weight forward. 4. Move hands up in a curve, palms up, and cross wrists in front of chest with right hand on outside and palms facing in; at same time draw right foot in and point toes to ground. 5-6. Spread arms out to rides, elbows slightly bent and palms facing out; at same time raise right knee and slowly straighten leg; kick with right heel and keep eyes on right hand.

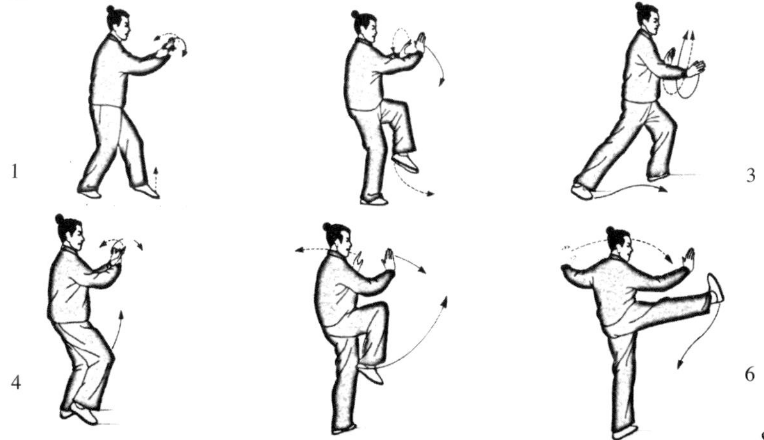

Striking Ears With Both Fists

1-2. Draw right leg back with knee still raised, at same time bring left hand forward next to right hand, drop hands beside right knee, palms up, and look ahead. 3-4. put right foot forward and step forward. Shift weight gradually to right leg, which should be bent, and keep left leg straight; at same time clench fists slowly and lower them first to sides and then up and forward at eye level. Keep fists facing each other at a distance of 10-20 cm (4-8 in) and keep eyes on right fist.

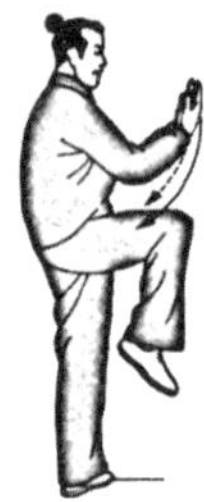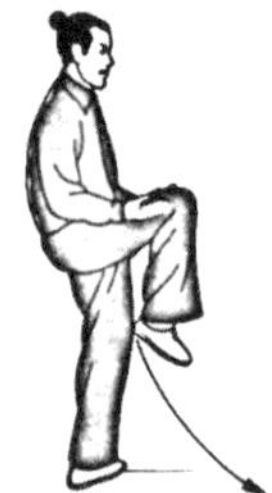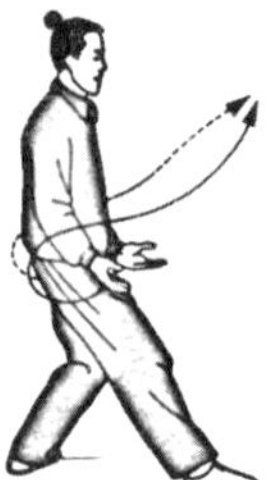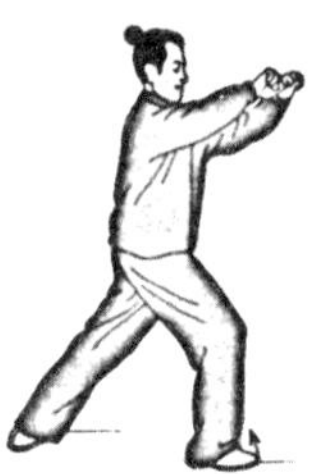

Kicking With the Left Heel

1. Bend left knee, shift weight to left leg and turn torso to left, toes of right foot raised and turned in. 2. At same time unclench fists and spread arms to sides, palms facing forward, eyes looking at left hand. 3-4. Shift weight onto right leg and draw left foot in, toes pointing to ground; at same time move hands down and up in a curve and cross wrists in front of chest with left hand on outside, palms facing in. 5-6. Spread arms out to sides, elbows slightly bent and palms facing out; at same time raise left knee and straighten leg slowly, kicking with left heel, eyes looking at left.

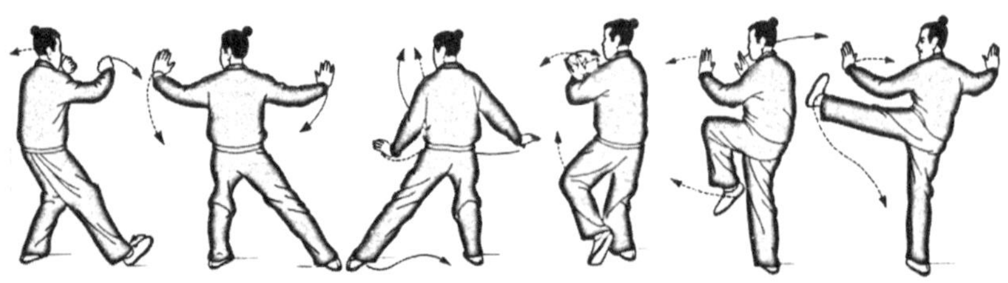

Section Six – Sweeping Down To Left On One Leg

1-2. Draw left leg back with knees still raised and turn torso to right; at same time hook right hand by bending wrist and move left hand up in a curve and down to front of right shoulder, palm facing in and eyes looking at right hand. 3. Bend right knee slowly, lower left leg and stretch it out to left. 4. While squatting down on right leg move left hand down in a curve, past inside of left leg, eyes looking at left hand. 5. Shift weight forward to left leg, which should be bent, and keep right leg straight; turn left toe out and right toe in as much as possible. At same time continue to stretch left hand forward, palm upright, and lower right hand, which should be hooked, and keep eyes on left hand. 6-7. Raise right knee down and stand on left leg; at same time raise right hand to eye level with elbow bent just above right knee and palm facing left. Lower left hand to hip, palm down, and look at right hand.

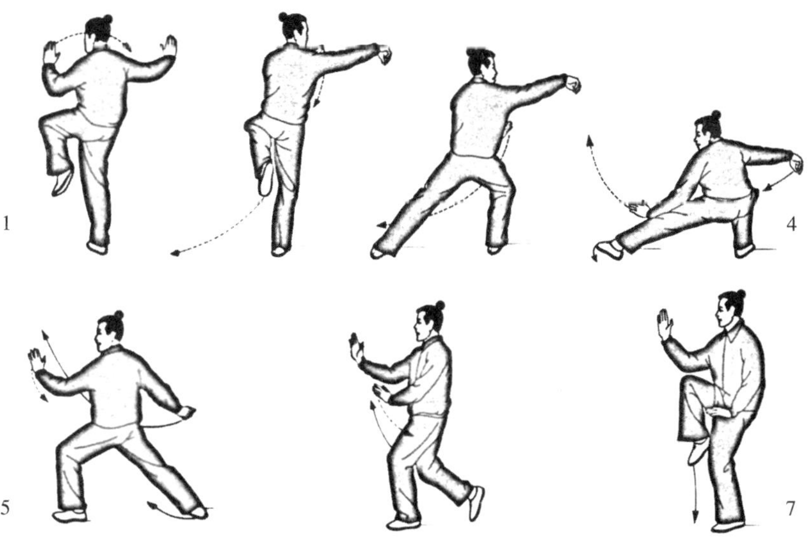

Sweeping Down To Right On One Leg

1-2. Place your right foot in front of your left foot, keeping right heel off ground, and pivoting on ball of left foot turn body to left. At same time raise left arm, hook left hand and move right hand to front of left shoulder, palm facing in and eyes on left hand. 3-4. Repeat steps 3-4 of Sweeping down to left on one leg, but in opposite direction. 5. Repeat step 5 of sweeping down to left on one leg, but in opposite direction. 6-7. Repeat steps 6-7 of sweeping down to left on one leg, but in opposite direction.

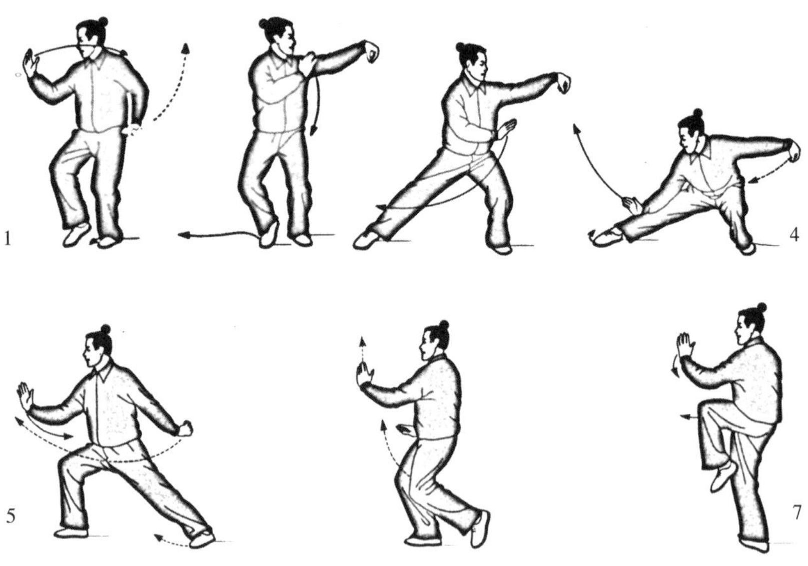

Section Seven – Passing The Shuttle To Left and Right

1-2. Turn body slightly to left and place left foot in front of right foot. Squat and lift right heel; at same time position hands in front of chest as though holding a ball, left hand above right hand. 3. Draw right foot next lo left foot with only toes touching ground and keep eyes on left arm. 4-6. Turn body lo right, step forward with right foot and keeping left leg straight, bend right knee, at same time lift right hand and hold it to right side of forehead, palm up. Lower left hand and push it forward until it reaches eye level, palm facing forward; keep eyes on left hand. 7-8. Shift your weight slightly back so that toes of your right foot turn out. Put weight on right leg and draw left foot beside right foot, left heel raised; at same time position hands in front of chest as though holding a ball, right hand above left hand, and keep eyes on right arm. 9-11. Repeat steps 4-6, but in opposite direction.

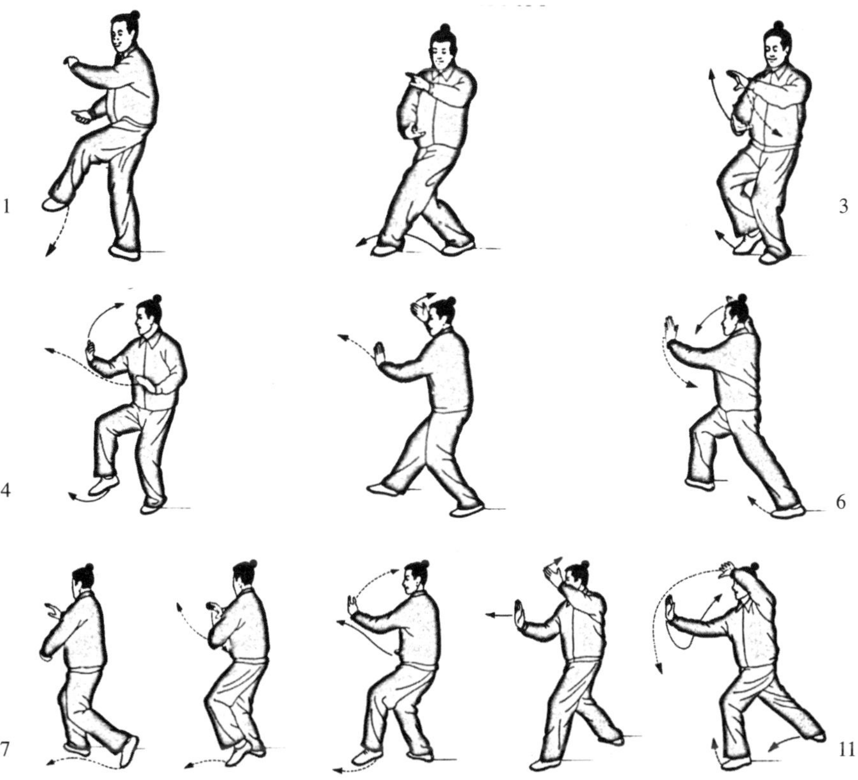

Needle At Sea Bottom

1-2. Take half a step forward with right foot, shift weight to right leg, lift left foot and point toes to ground; at same time turn body slightly to right and move right hand down in a curve and up to side of right ear. Turn body to left, drop right hand forward, palm facing left; at same time lower left hand forward, then down in a curve and rest it at side of left hip, palm down; keep eyes on right hand.

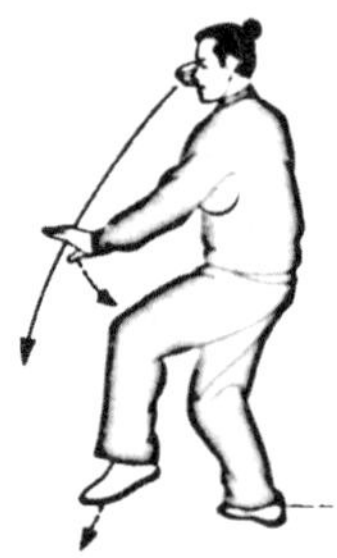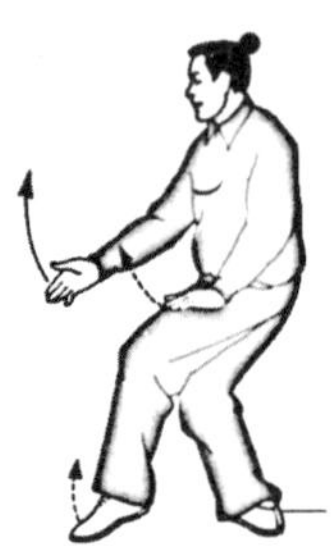

Dodge With The Arm

1. Turn torso slightly to right and step forward with left foot, keep right leg straight and bend left knee. 2. At same time raise right hand, bend elbow and hold hand at right side of forehead, palm up. 3. At same time lift left hand and push it forward at chest level with palm facing front; keep eyes on left hand.

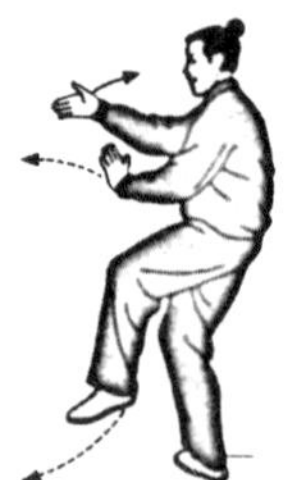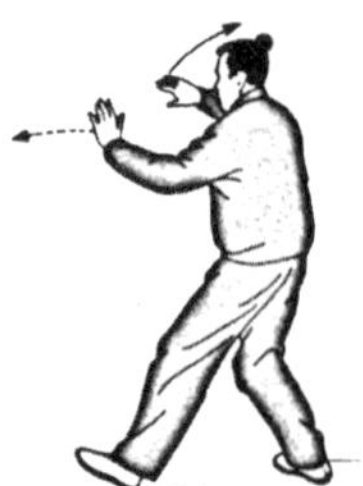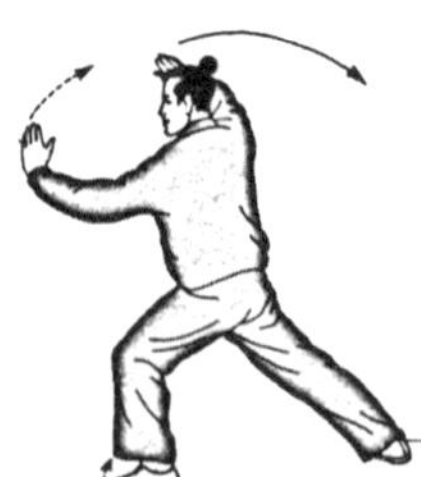

Section Eight – Turn To Strike, Parry and Punch

1. Lower torso, shift weight onto right leg and turn body to right with toes of left foot lifted off ground; at same time lift left hand and hold it in front of forehead with palm facing out. 2. Shift weight back to left leg, turn body slightly to right and move right hand down in a curve and hold it in front of left rib cage, palm down, keep eyes looking to right. 3-4. Turn body to right, draw right leg back and step forward again; at same time flick right fist over to right, crossing chest, palm up, and drop left hand beside hip, palm down. Drop your right foot firmly on the ground, with its toes turned out, and keep your eyes on your right fist. 5-6. Shift weight onto right leg and step forward with left foot, at same time push forward with left hand and draw right fist back to waist, palm up, eyes looking at left hand. 7. Keep right leg straight, bend left knee and punch forward with right fist, thumb facing up; hold inside of right elbow with left hand, keeping eyes on right fist.

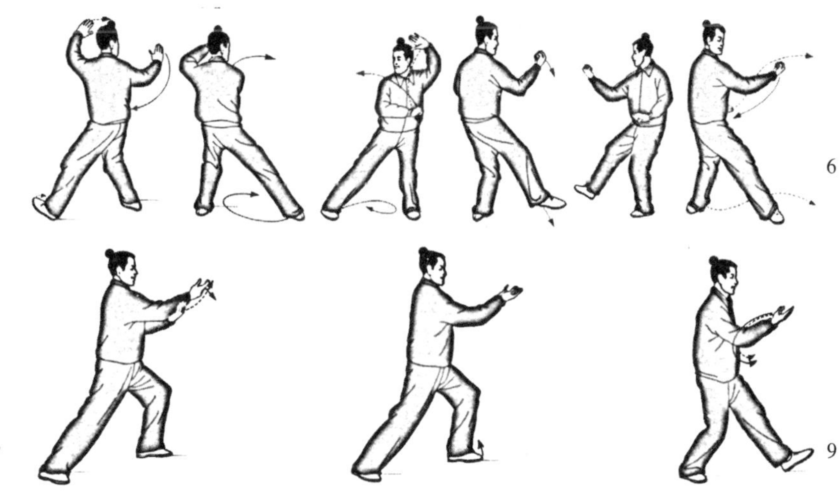

Withdraw And Push

1-2. Stretch left hand out, passing it under right wrist, and unclench right fist so that palms face up. 3. Lower elbows slowly and draw hands back, at same time lower torso, shift weight to right leg and lift toes of left foot off ground. 4-6. Turn palms over and push forward with hands from abdomen up to shoulder level. At same time keeping right leg straight, bend left leg, put weight on it and look straight ahead.

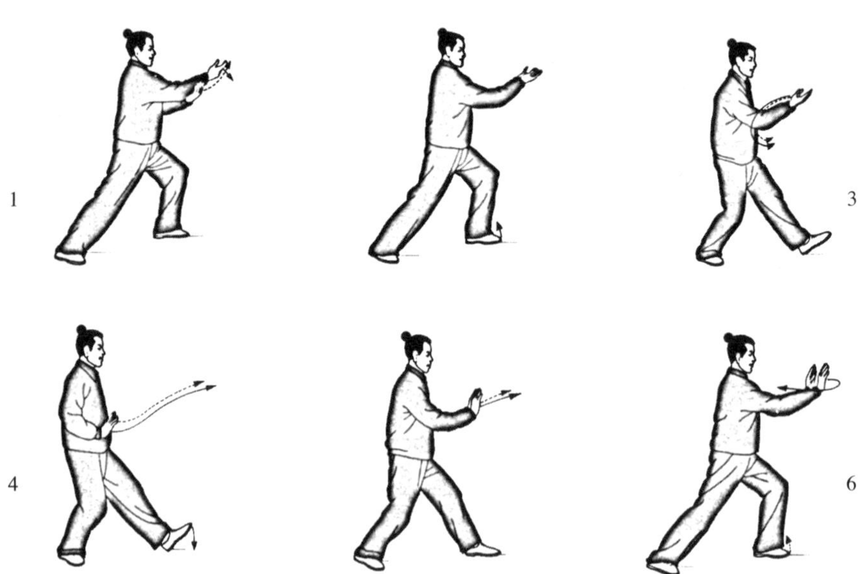

Crossing Arms

1-2. Bend right knee, shift weight to right leg, lift left foot and turn toes in, at same time turn body to right and stretch right arm up so that palms are facing out. Bend elbows, slightly and keep eyes on right hand. 3-4. Shift weight slowly to left leg and draw right foot back so that it is parallel with left foot, but shoulder-width apart. At same time bring hands down and up to shoulder level and cross arms, right hand on outside, palms facing in, and look straight ahead.

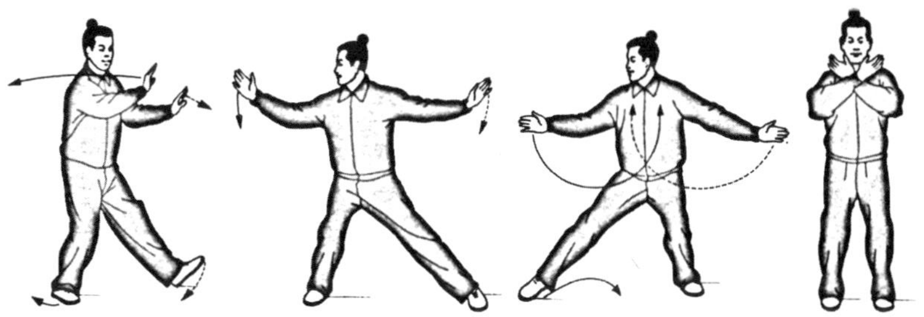

Conclusion

1-3. Turn palms over to face out, slowly drop arms to side, palms facing down, and look straight ahead. When lowering arms relax whole body, breathe out slowly, bring left foot next to right foot and stand straight.

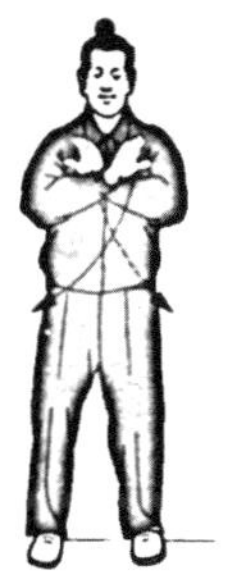 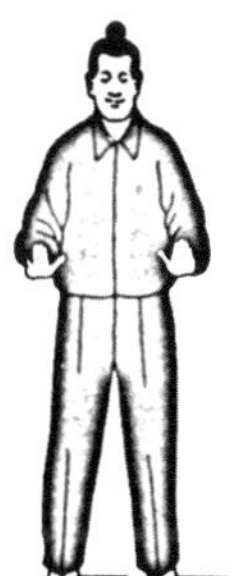 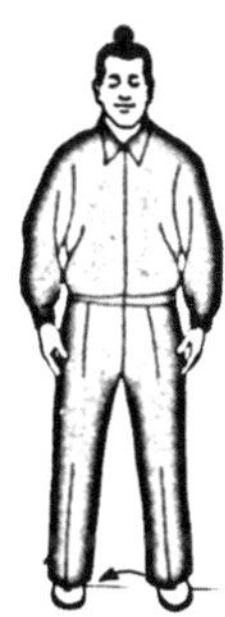

Chinese Saber

To practice the Chinese Saber or Taiji Sword correctly, the first thing a practitioner must be able to do is to have a flexible body and wrist so that the sword (for safety proposes I recommend using a wooden sword when family members are practicing, to minimize any potential injuries) and the body will coordinate and move in unity.

The second thing is that the intent should direct each movement so that all the movements have varies applications, speed and accuracy. The third thing is to have spirit and natural breathing in each movement. In usage, it also emphasizes the concepts of sticking and adhering, running and following. The Taiji Sword practitioner must execute all the movements in an even, soft, continuous and smooth manner. All the movements are initiated by the waist, controlled by the wrist, with the upper and lower parts of the body coordinated so that when one part of the body moves, all parts follow. When one part stops, all stop. Therefore, all the movements are very light, speedy, flexible, nimble, and stable. People often describe these kinds of motions as like a "swimming dragon and flying phoenix."

When practicing the sword the actions employed are chopping, stirring, stroking and stabbing. The techniques are finely linked together. One is drawing forth (of opponents attack) and one is striking; one is flourishing and one is presentation. The body follows the movements of the sword which circles the body and can be seen on every direction. Lithe and graceful, surprising and subtle; body and sword are as one. Like a Spiritual Dragon, speeding like an arrow, or a male phoenix soaring and circling in the air. Remember to:

to chop
to stir divert and slash in one continuous movement
to stroke subtle circular diversion
to stab/pierce
to draw forth diverting upwards with a whipping action
to lift an upward diversion
to sweep across horizontal diversion followed by thrust
to invert diverting to the side, sword pointed down

Holding the Sword in Your Left Hand - Hold guard with thumb pointing down, index finger stretched, and other fingers pointing up Make sure the sword is close to the body and parallel to left forearm with blade facing away from the body.

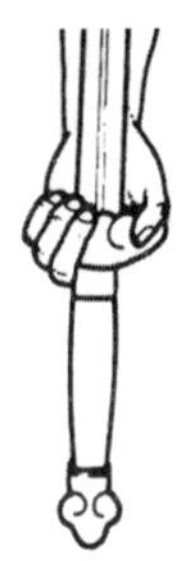

Holding the Sward in Your Right Hand - Hold handle with thumb and index finger, keep other 3 fingers in a more relaxed and flexible position and control movement of sword with base of palm. An alternative way to hold sword in right hand is to tighten middle finger, ring finger and thumb around handle and to relax the index and little fingers.

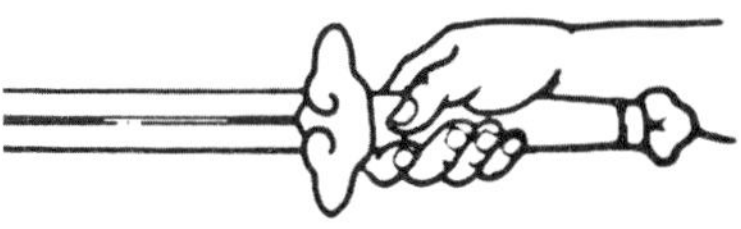

Sword Fingers - The sword finger is an essential movement in the performance, it can help the sword practitioner to concentrate the mind and balance of the body. The body of the sword should be spiritual and energized. The evaluation of the sword is to follow by the eyes to show the direction of the movement. If the tassel twists around the sword or the hand, which means the movement is not correct or the wrong strength is used. Stretch your index finger and middle finger and bend your little finger, thumb and ring finger into your palm of your hand.

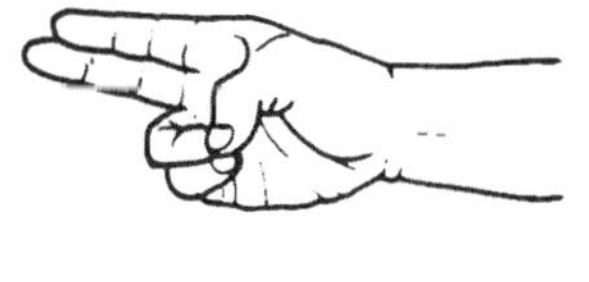

Preparation

1.Breathe in; stand at ease, keeping your body straight with your feet shoulder-width apart, toes pointing forward and arms hanging naturally at your side. Hold your sword, pointing straight up, in your left hand, and your right hand palm facing your body, fingers pointing down, looking straight ahead and relax your shoulders. 2. Breathe out; raise your arms slowly to your shoulders, form right hand into sword fingers, palms of both hands facing down, and hold your sword facing down, and hold the sword parallel to the ground. 3-4. Breathe in; turn your torso slightly to the right, shifting your weight to the right leg; lower body, turn torso to left, lift leg, step to the left and, keeping right leg straight, bend your left knee. At the same time move your left hand to the right and follow Turing of the torso downward in a curve to the left; hold hand at your left hip with sword pointing straight up. Simultaneously drop your sword fingers, then bring them up and forward and point them straight ahead at eye level. Keep your eyes on the sword fingers. Breathe out; come back into standing position. Repeat this cycle 4 times.

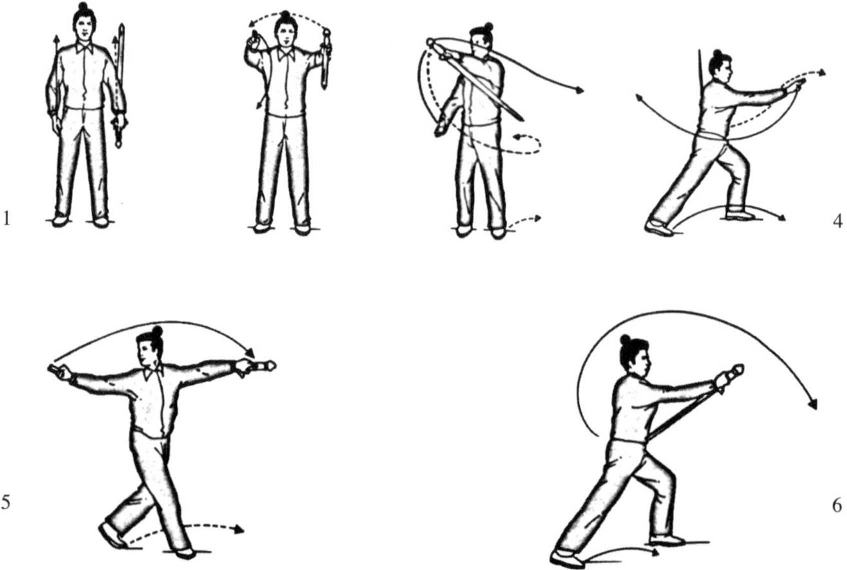

Section One

Point and Thrust

1. Breathe in; come into a standing position. Hold your sword in your right hand move it up and down in a curving motion. Point your sword forward and take hold of your right wrist with your left hand which is formed into sword fingers; while at the same time bring your right foot forward so that your feet are together and knees are bent, keeping your eyes on the tip of your sword. 2. Breathe out; step back with your right foot and turn your torso to the right, then draw your left foot back with the heel off the ground; while at the same time turn your right wrist over and bring your right hand over behind you, drawing a circle with the tip of your sword. Follow your sword with your left hand formed into sword fingers and rest them on your right shoulder; keeping your eyes resting on the tip of your sword. 3. Breathe in; turning your torso to the left, lift your left knee and stand on your right foot, while at the same time raise your right hand and pass the sword over your head with a thrusting movement. Stretch left hand, formed into sword fingers, forward and keep eyes on fingers. Breathe out; turn your body to the left, shifting your body weight onto your left leg, and bring right foot parallel with your left foot, but shoulder-width apart; while at the same time take hold of the sword with your left hand and drop it naturally to your side, keeping the blade of the sword parallel with your forearm, sword pointing upward. Draw your right hand back and up in a curve and hang it by your side. Relax your whole body and look straight ahead. Repeat cycle 4 times.

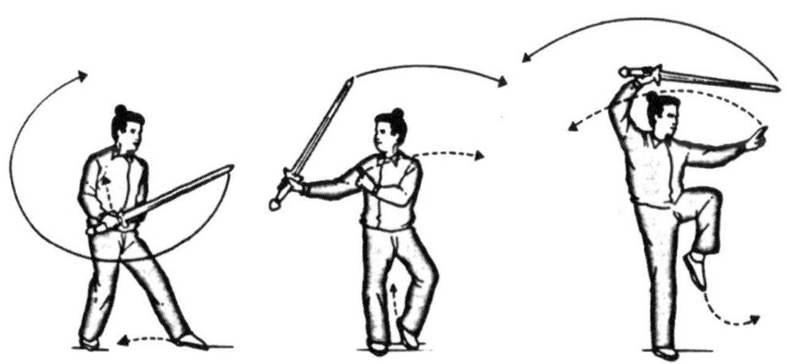

Sweep and Take to the Right

1. Breathe in; turn your torso to the right and make a chopping movement, bringing the sword back and behind to your right and keep your arm straight. Hold your right wrist with your left hand formed into sword fingers, while at the same time keep your left leg straight, bend you're your right knee, lowering your left leg and stretch it backward; keeping your eyes on the tip of the

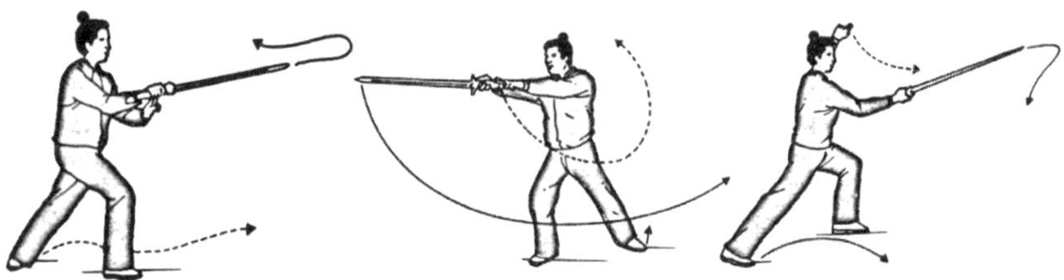

sword. 2. Breath out; turn your torso to the left and swing your left hand forward into sword fingers over and down and up in a curve and hold above your head, palm facing up. At the same time sweep your sword in the same direction. While making sweeping movements and following turning of the body, shift your weight onto your left foot and keep your right leg straight, bend left knee; keeping your eyes on the tip of the sword. 3. Breathe in; lift your right leg, step forward and keeping your left leg straight, bend your right knee; while at the same time stretch your right hand, turn sword-holding palm downward and slowly withdraw sword and elbow slightly bent in front of right ribs. Drop your left hand formed into sword fingers to right wrist and keep eyes on tip of the sword. 4. Breathe out; stretch your right hand forward, turning your sword-holding palm upward, slowly withdraw your sword with elbow slightly bent in front of your left ribs; while at the same time bring your left hand formed into sword fingers down past your left ribs and up in a curve to the left of your forehead, with the palm up. At the same time step forward with your left foot and, keeping right leg straight, bend your left knee; keeping your eyes on the tip of the sword. 5. Breathe out; bring your right foot beside your left foot, with your heel off the ground, dropping your left hand formed into sword fingers onto your right wrist. 6. Breathe in; turning your body to the left and bring your sword

back and behind in a curve to your left, turning your wrist up. 7. Breathe out; swing your left hand formed into sword fingers over your head, palm up; while at the same time make a chopping movement with your sword to your right, step forward with your right foot and lift your left knee high, keeping your eyes on the tip of your sword. Breathe out; turn your body to the left, shifting your body weight onto your left leg, and bring right foot parallel with your left foot, but shoulder-width apart; while at the same time take hold of the sword with your left hand and drop it naturally to your side, keeping the blade of the sword parallel with your forearm, sword pointing upward. Draw your right hand back and up in a curve and hang it by your side. Relax your whole body and look straight ahead. Repeat this cycle 4 times.

Retreat, Whip and Thrust to One Foot

1. Breathe in; drop your left foot behind your back, with your knee bent, draw your right foot back half a step, heel off the ground; while at the same time make a whipping movement, bring your sword handle close to your left ribs, with the tip of your sword pointing outward. Drop your left hand formed in sword fingers onto your sword handle. 2. Breathe out; step forward with your right foot and left knee high; while at the same time thrust your sword up, and palm up. Keeping your left hand formed into sword fingers on the handle of your sword keep your eyes on the tip of the sword. 3. Breathe out; come back into standing position raising your arms slowly to your shoulders, form right hand into sword fingers, palms of both hands facing down, and hold your sword facing down, and hold the sword parallel to the ground. Repeat this cycle 4 times.

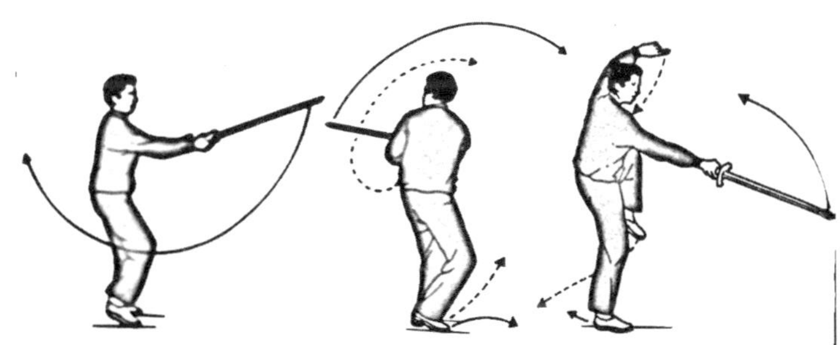

Section Two

Cut and Thrust

1. Breathe in; drop your left foot behind your back and draw your right foot slightly back, with your heel off the ground; while at the same time following the turning of your body, first to the left and then to the right, make a downward cutting movement with your sword, it tip at the knee level. Bring your left hand formed into sword fingers down and up in a curve to top left corner of your forehead, palm up, and look straight ahead. 2. Breathe out; step back with your right foot, draw the left foot back then step forward to the left and, keeping your right leg straight, bend your left knee. At the same time following the movement of your body bring your sword to shoulder level, drawing the sword back, lowering it and making a forward thrusting movement to your left, palm up; while at the same time drop your left hand formed in sword fingers down in a curve to your right, raise them in a curve to the top of the left corner of the forehead, palm up, and keep your eyes on the tip of the sword. 3. Breathe out; come back into standing position raising your arms slowly to your shoulders, form right hand into sword fingers, palms of both hands facing down, and hold your sword facing down, and hold the sword parallel to the ground. Repeat this cycle 4 times.

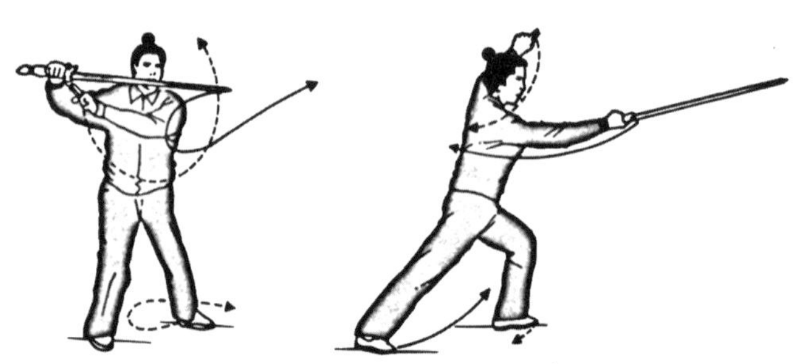

Turn Around and Shrink Back

1. Breathe in; pivoting on your left heel, turn your body to the right and lift your right foot to touch your left leg; while at the same time draw your right hand back to your chest, palm up. Keeping the blade of your sword parallel to the ground, dropping your left hand formed in sword fingers to rest on your right wrist, keeping your eyes on the tip of your sword. 2. Breathe out; turning your body to the right, drop your right foot to the ground and keeping your left leg straight, bend your right knee; at the same time following the turning of your body, stretch your right arm with the sword, exerting force on the outside of the blade and turn the tip of the sword up and keep your palm down. Rest your left hand formed in sword fingers on your right wrist and keep your eyes on the tip of your sword. 3. Breathe in; lift and lower your left leg, drawing your right foot back next to your left foot, heel off the ground, while shifting your weight onto your left foot; while at the same time stretch your left arm with the sword, palm up, except force on the outside of the blade and turn the tip of the sword up. Move your left hand formed in sword fingers down and back in a curve and then return them to rest on the right wrist keeping your eyes on the tip of the sword. 4. Breathe out; come back into standing position raising your arms slowly to your shoulders, form right hand into sword fingers, palms of both hands facing down, and hold your sword facing down, and hold the sword parallel to the ground. Repeat this cycle 4 times.

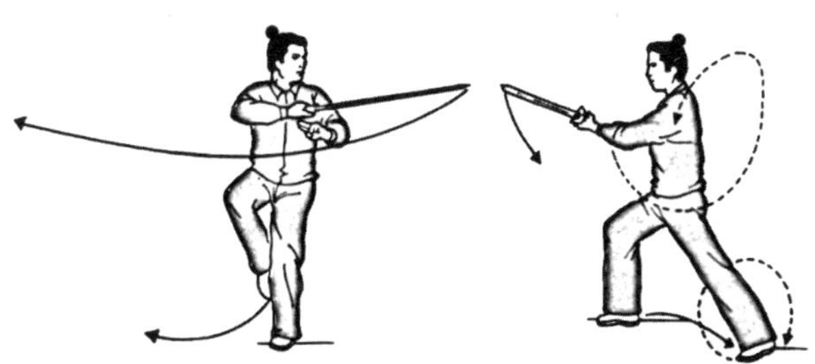

Lifting Knee and Holding Sword

1. Breathe in; step back with your right foot and follow with your left foot, heel off the ground; while at the same time separate your hands moving your left hand with the sword to the right and the right hand formed in sword fingers to the left, both palms down. 2. Breathe out; drop the foot to the ground and lift the right knee high; while at the same time open the left hand to hold the right

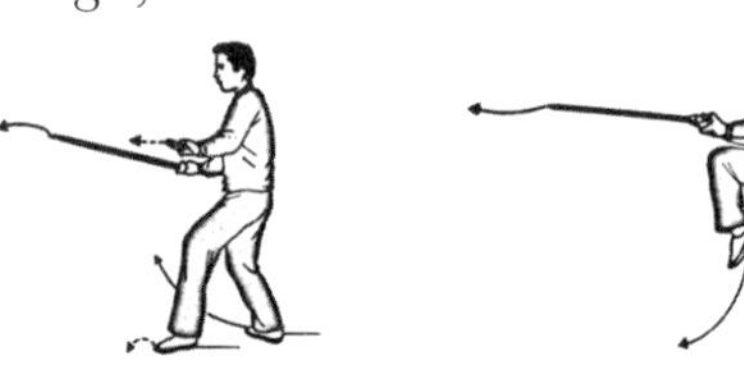

hand and bring the sword handle toward your chest, arms slightly bent, sword pointing forward and eyes looking ahead. 3. Breathe out; come back into standing position raising your arms slowly to your shoulders, form right hand into sword fingers, palms of both hands facing down, and hold your sword facing down, and hold the sword parallel to the ground. Repeat this cycle 4 times.

Thrust

1. Breathe in; lower your right foot, shift your weight forward; while at the same time thrust your sword forward with force. 2. Breathe out; stamp your toes of the right foot hard, step forward with your left foot and quickly raise your right heel to the side of the left leg; while at the same time separate and lower your hands to your sides, palms down, left hand formed into sword fingers, eyes looking straight ahead. 3. Breathe in; stepping forward with your right foot and, keeping your left leg straight, bend right knee; while at the same time thrust your sword forward, palm up, eyes looking at tip of your sword. Bring the left hand formed into sword fingers over your head in a backward and upward curve, palm up. 4. Breathe out; come back into standing position raising your arms slowly to your shoulders, form right hand into sword fingers, palms of both hands facing down, and hold your sword facing down, and hold the sword parallel to the ground. Repeat this cycle 4 times.

Provoke to Left and to Right

1. Breathe in; turn your torso to the left and shift your body weight onto your left leg. Draw your right foot back half a step and, with your weight shifted onto the right leg, turn your body to the right and step forward with your left foot, heel off the ground. 2. Breathe out; at the same time, follow turning of the body, make a provoking movement with your right forearm turned inward and palm facing outward, move your sword in a curve down to the left and then up in a curve to the right. Stop your sword handle at the level of your eyes and follow the movement of the right wrist with your left hand formed into a sword finger gesture and keep your eyes on the tip of your sword. 3. Breathe in; come back into standing position. 4. Breathe out; turn torso to your right and draw your sword up and down to the right in a curve, both your palms facing out. Put left foot down, step to your left with your right foot and keeping your left leg straight, bend your right knee, while at the same time continue with provoking movement of the sword down and up in a curve to the left; turning your right forearm out with your palm facing out. Keep your sword at shoulder level, raising your left hand formed into a sword finger gesture above your head and keep your eyes on the tip of your sword. 5. Breathe out; come back into standing position raising your arms slowly to your shoulders, form right hand into sword fingers, palms of both hands facing down, and hold your sword facing down, and hold the sword parallel to the ground. Repeat this cycle 4 times.

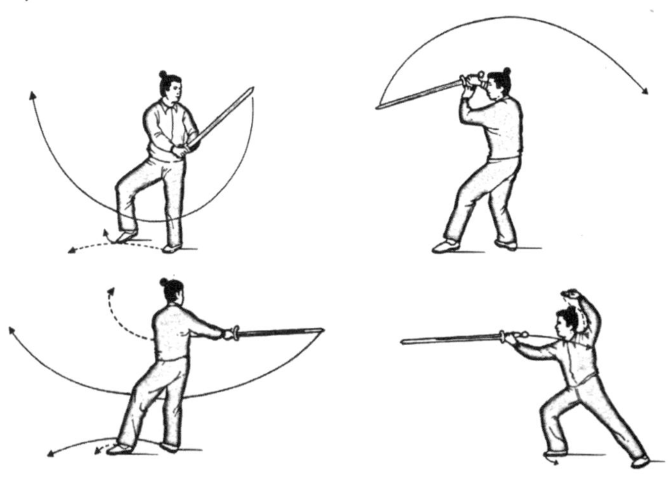

Section Three

Turn Left to Lash

1. Breathe in; turn your body to the left, shifting your weight backward, straighten your right leg and bend your left knee slightly; while at the same time draw your sword back to the front of the chest, with your left hand formed into sword fingers touching your right wrist. 2. Breathe out; continue to turn to the left with your left knee bent, making a chopping movement to your left with your sword, keeping your eyes on the tip of your sword. 3. Breathe in; bend your right knee slightly, shifting your weight back to the right leg and draw the left foot back, with the heel off the ground; while at the same time make a lashing movement, pulling the sword back to your right hip; draw the left hand formed into sword fingers back to your chest, stretch your fingers forward again, keeping your eyes on them. 4. Breathe out; come back into standing position raising your arms slowly to your shoulders, form right hand into sword fingers, palms of both hands facing down, and hold your sword facing down, and hold the sword parallel to the ground. Repeat this cycle 4 times.

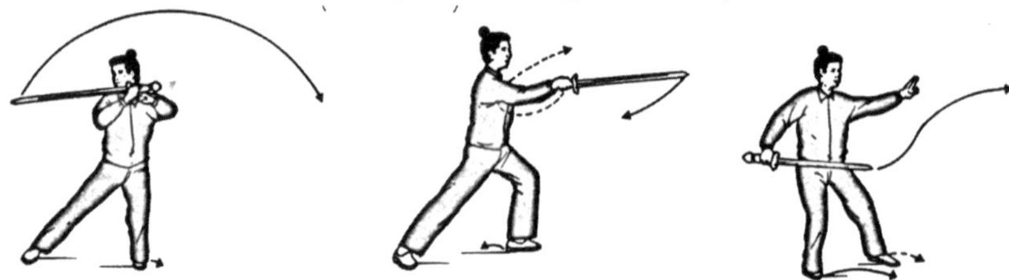

Parry to Left and Right

1. Breathe in; put your left foot down, move your right foot forward and stand straight with your feet together; while at the same time open your left hand to the right hand and thrust your sword forward, palms up, keeping your eyes on the tip of your sword. 2. Breathe out; pull the sword back, keep your left hand formed into sword fingers at right wrist and turn your torso to the right. Follow turning of your body to the left and make a parrying movement with the sword, drawing a backward, downward and forward curve to your left, with your right forearm turned

outward. Raise your left hand formed into a sword finger gesture above your head; while at the same time step forward to the left with your left foot and keeping the right leg straight, bend your left knee and keep your eyes on the movement of your sword. 3. Breathe out: shift weight slightly backward while turning your torso to the left with your left toes slanting out, then turn your torso to the right, step forward with right foot and, keeping left your leg straight , bend your right knee; at the same time parry with your sword to the left in a downward and forward curve, turning your right forearm in, palm facing out; at the same time return the left hand formed into a sword finger gesture to the right wrist,

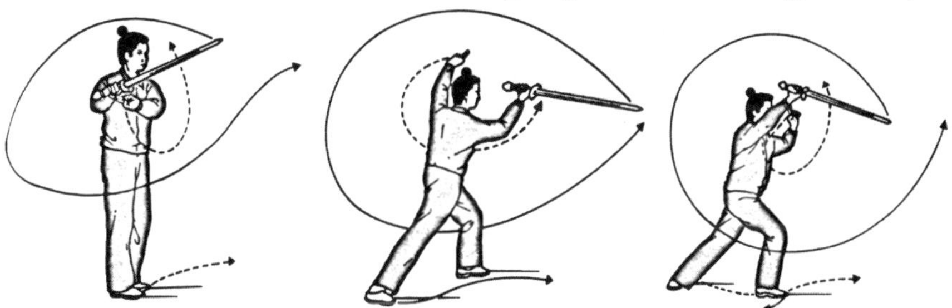

keeping your eyes on the movements of the sword. 4. Breathe out; come back into standing position raising your arms slowly to your shoulders, form right hand into sword fingers, palms of both hands facing down, and hold your sword facing down, and hold the sword parallel to the ground. Repeat this cycle 4 times.

Parry to left and Stab

1. Breathe in; shift your body weight slightly backward while turning your right toes out, step forward with your left foot and, keeping the right leg straight, bend your left knee and turn your torso to the left; while at the same time parry with the sword in a backward, downward and forward curve, turn your right forearm out and raise your left hand formed into a sword finger gesture above your head. 2. Breathe out; turn your body to the right and cross your right leg over to the left, lifting left heel off the ground; at the same lower the tip of your sword, drop your left hand formed into sword fingers to the right wrist, spread your arms out and make a stabbing movement with your sword to your right, palm

facing forward, eyes following the tip of the sword. 3. Breathe in; turning your body to the left, step forward with your left foot

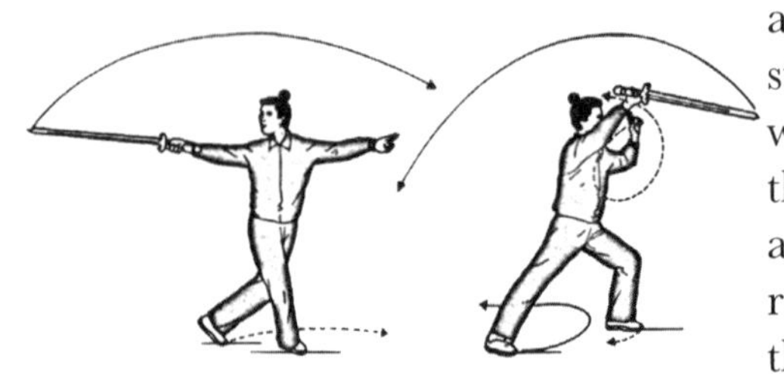

and keeping your right leg straight, bend the left knee; while at the same time bring the tip of the sword down in a curve to the left with your right forearm turned in and the palm facing out; rest your left hand formed into sword fingers on the right wrist and keep your eyes on the tip of your sword. 4. Breathe out; come back into standing position raising your arms slowly to your shoulders, form right hand into sword fingers, palms of both hands facing down, and hold your sword facing down, and hold the sword parallel to the ground. Repeat this cycle 4 times.

Turn Left and Chop

1. Breathe in; shift your weight onto your right foot while turning your toes of your left foot in, lift your right leg and shift your weight onto the left leg. Turn your body to the right, stepping forward with your right foot and, keeping your left leg straight, bend your right knee; while at the same time with the force of your right wrist, make a chopping movement with your sword in the same direction as the body is turning; lift your left hand formed in sword fingers above your head, in an upward and downward curve. Keep your eyes on the tip of your sword. 2. Breathe out; lift your left foot while turning your torso to the left, put your left foot down and lift your right foot up and put it down in front of your left foot with the heel off the ground; while at the same time draw your sword up in a curve and point it forward and down. Form your left hand into sword fingers and bring them around in a circle to rest on your right wrist; keeping your eyes on the tip of your sword. 3. Breathe out; come back into standing position raising your arms slowly to your shoulders, form right hand into sword fingers, palms of both hands facing down, and hold your sword facing down, and hold the sword parallel to the ground. Repeat this cycle 4 times.

Fourth Section

Stand on One Foot to Hang and Chop

1. Breathe in; bring your right foot behind your left foot and, pivoting on the balls of both feet, turn your body to the right and raise your left knee; while at the same time draw a circle with your sword (left, down and up) and hold the sword up to the right slightly above the level of your head. Form the left hand into sword fingers, hold the left hand close to the right wrist and look straight ahead. 2. Breathe out; drop the left foot to your side and turn your body to the left, knees crossed and bent, raise the right heel off the ground; while at the same time make a hanging movement with your sword to the rear, keep the left hand formed into sword fingers next to your right wrist and follow tip the sword with your eyes. 3. Breathe in; make a chopping movement with your sword toward the right; lift your left hand formed into sword fingers above your head and at the same time step forward with your right foot and, keeping your left leg straight, with right knee bent, keeping your eyes on the tip of the sword. 4. Breathe out; come back into standing position raising your arms slowly to your shoulders, form right hand into sword fingers, palms of both hands facing down, and hold your sword facing down, and hold the sword parallel to the ground. Repeat this cycle 4 times.

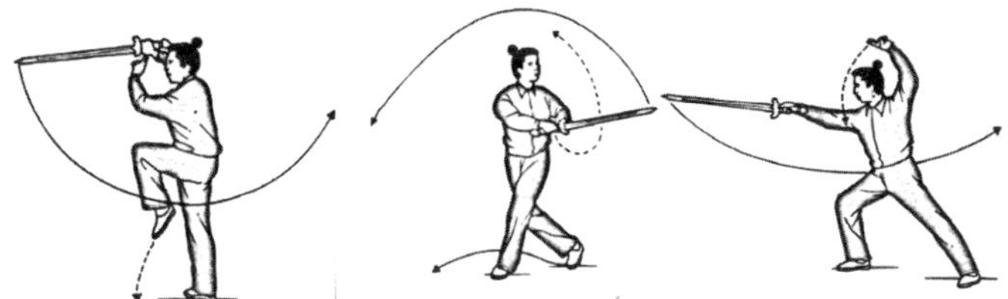

Provoke Chop and Strike

1. Breathe in; shift your body weight slightly backward and turn body to the left, knees crossed, and lift your left heel off the ground; at the same make a provoking movement with your sword in a downward curve and up to your right; dropping your left hand formed in sword fingers to your right shoulder and keep your eyes on the tip of your sword. 2. Breathe out; step forward with your left foot, turn your body to your left then step forward with your right foot, with the heel off the ground; while at the same time make a forward chopping movement with the sword first backward then forward, keeping the tip of the sword level with your knee. Move your left hand formed in sword fingers down in a curve and up to rest on your right forearm; keep eyes on the tip of your sword..3. Breathe in; turn your body to the right and take a large step with your right foot and keeping your left leg straight, bend your right knee; while at the same time make a striking movement with your sword back and upward following turning of your body and hold the tip of the sword above eye level. Point your left hand formed into a sword finger gesture toward your left, keep eyes on the tip of your sword. 4. Breathe out; come back into standing position raising your arms slowly to your shoulders, form right hand into sword fingers, palms of both hands facing down, and hold your sword facing down, and hold the sword parallel to the ground. Repeat this cycle 4 times.

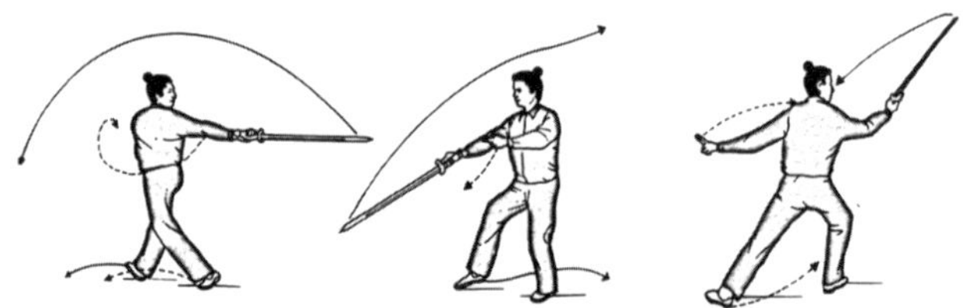

Step Forward to Thrust and to Whip

1. Breathe in; lift your left leg and bring it down close to your right leg; while at the same time turn your right palm over and bring your sword to the front of the right shoulder, pointing to your left; bring your left hand formed in a sword finger gesture to your right shoulder and look straight ahead. 2. Breathe out; turn your body around and toward the left, placing your left foot on the ground, step forward with your right foot and keeping your left leg straight, bend your right knee; while at the same time as turning your body thrust your sword forward with force, palm up. Raise your left hand formed into a sword finger gesture above your head. 3. Breathe in; shift your body weight backward and draw your right foot back beside your left foot, with the heel off the ground; while at the same time bend your right elbow and draw back the sword, palm facing in and sword handle near your left ribs. Drop your left hand formed into a sword finger gesture onto the handle of the sword and keep your eyes on the tip of the sword. 4. Breathe out; come back into standing position raising your arms slowly to your shoulders, form right hand into sword fingers, palms of both hands facing down, and hold your sword facing down, and hold the sword parallel to the ground. Repeat this cycle 4 times.

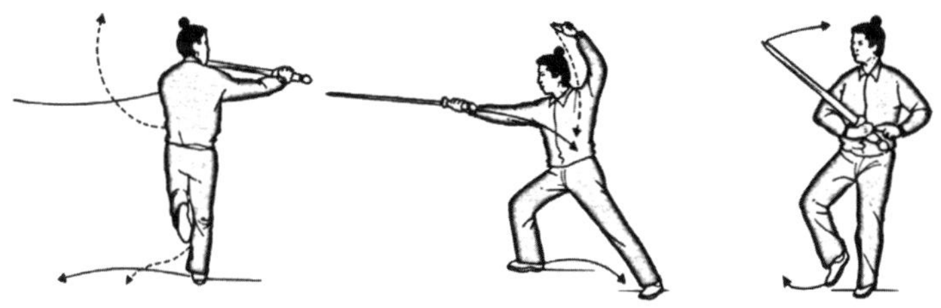

To Swipe with Body Revolving

1. Breathe in; lift your right foot and step forward with your toes turned out; while at the same time turn your torso slightly to the right and stretch your arms out so that your sword is positioned in front of your chest. 2. Breathe out; shift your body weight onto the right leg and keep turning to your right; move your left foot in front of your right foot, toes pointing toward each other, toes pointing toward each other; pivoting on the ball of your left foot, continue to turn your body to right until your right foot is a step behind your left foot; draw left foot back half step, toes pointing toward the ground. At the same time following revolving of your body, make a sweeping movement with your sword parallel to the ground and separate your hands with palms facing down.

Breathe in; come back into standing position raising your arms slowly to your shoulders, form right hand into sword fingers, palms of both hands facing down, and hold your sword facing down, and hold the sword parallel to the ground. Repeat this cycle 4 times.

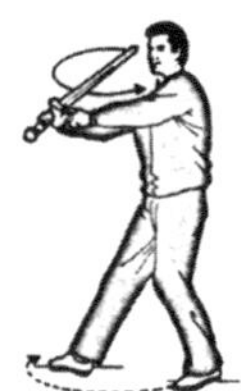 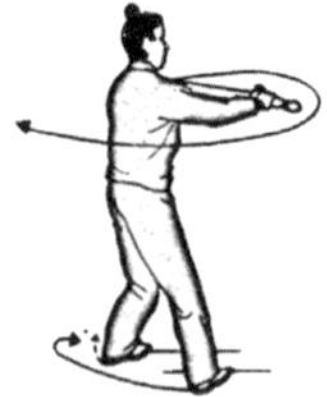 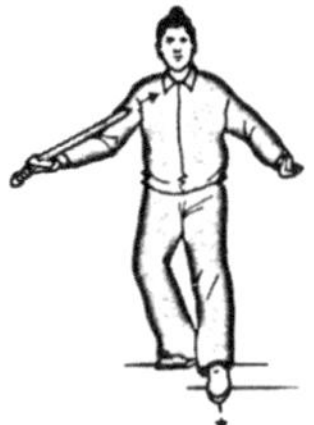

Thrust Forward

1. Breathe in; take a half step forward with your left foot and keeping your right leg straight bend your left knee; while at the same time make a stabbing movement with your sword, thrusting it straight forward. Keep your left hand formed in a sword finger gesture resting on your right wrist and look straight ahead. 2. Breathe out; shift; shift your body weight backward and turn body to your right; while at the same time draw back your sword, palm facing in, and put your left hand on the sword hand guard, palm facing your right palm. Keep your eyes on the tip of the sword. 3. Breathe in; turn your body to the left, shifting your body weight onto your left leg, and bring right foot parallel with your left foot, but shoulder-width apart; while at the same time take hold of the sword with your left hand and drop it naturally to your side, keeping the blade of the sword parallel with your forearm, sword pointing upward. Draw your right hand back and up in a curve and hang it by your side. Relax your whole body and look straight ahead.

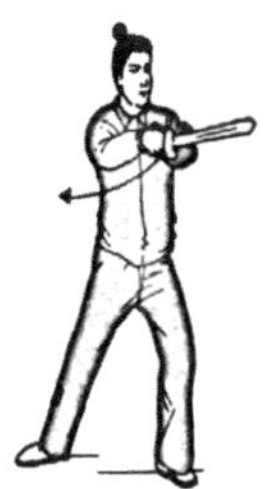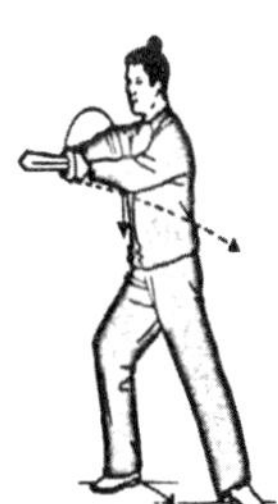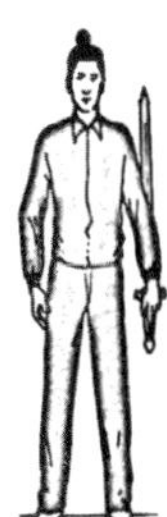

Pushing Hands or Tui Shou Movements

Most people who have heard of Tai Chi know it as a gentle, flowing set of movements that senior citizens do in the park on Sunday mornings. At first glance, it doesn't even appear to be a martial art, in that each person is doing the same movements without coming in contact with anyone else, like some sort of slow-motion, silent line dance. The solo form, however, is just one aspect of Tai Chi that can be practiced by everyone in the family. This sequence of postures is designed to strengthen the legs, improve posture, balance, and circulation, and teach the basic principles of shifting weight, relaxing, and remaining rooted. For all its benefits, though, this aspect of Tai Chi is just the beginning for serious practitioners. What many Tai Chi enthusiasts find most interesting about the art is a two-person exercise known as push hands (sometimes referred to as "pushing hands, or Tui Shou.

Tui means "to push" and shou means "hands". So, tui shou means "pushing hands". But this term is not very exact. In the internal martial arts we are not pushing with our hands - each movement is produced by the whole body. We are using coordinated whole body power which is known as hun yuan li (or nei jin). And much more, tui shou is not only about pushing. We also strike with different parts of the body. Basically you can issue the force with hand, elbow, shoulder, foot, knee, hip or head.

Tui shou is the practice of "pushing hands", where we maintain and refine the principles of Taiji while practicing with a partner. It provides an opportunity to improve our sensitivity, and to understand better the meaning of Taiji by spontaneously and creatively, and martial applications of the Taiji form. Through the practice, we can begin to see that Taiji is more than a martial art so it can become a form of communication that is universal.

Pushing hands can be practiced in a variety of ways and is consequently accessible to anybody of any age. The soft way is the most well known, and is the best way to practice for health and to realize the subtle communications between practitioners. It also allows martial techniques to naturally arise, safely and using a minimum of strength, reducing the chance of injuries or tensions.

110

Once the body and mind have properly integrated the principles, pushing hands can then be practiced in a more dynamic fashion, with progressively more emphasis on martial efficiency. It still remains a soft practice, but it is done with a higher level of intensity. When practicing Push Hands be aware of the following:

In motion, move like a thundering wave.
When still, be like a mountain.
Rising up, be like a monkey.
Land swiftly and lightly like a bird.
Be steady like a rooster on one leg.
One's stance is as firm as a pine tree, yet expresses motion.
Spin swiftly and circularly like a wheel.
Bend and flex like a bow.
Waft gracefully like a leaf in the wind.
Sink like a heavy piece of metal.
Prey like a watchful, gliding eagle.
Accelerate like a gusty wind.

Posture

Head: Held naturally as being supported by cotton from the centre of the crown. Tongue resting on the roof of the month. Eyes level following the dominant limbs. Neck: Erect, without tension. Shoulders: Relaxed, soft and sloping. Elbows: Always lowered and natural, never lift above the wrist. Chest: Relaxed, never puffed out in army fashion. Do not slump shoulders and collapse the chest. Back: Spine erect, pelvis tilted forward, relaxed. Waist: Soft, flexible, relaxed and sunken. Bottom: Tucked in. Legs: Firm and solid, feet rooted, knees not locked.

Method of Moving and Training

When practising Taijiquan, the body should remain relaxed and natural. The movements should be slow, smooth and light. Though movements should be agile and light, they should remain centred and rooted. Movement should contain the principle of spirals and arcs, co-ordination and continuity. Mind involvement is implicit in the instruction 'the mind leads the movements', a meditative stillness in motion in degrees is illustrated in levels of attainment. Breathing should remain natural, deep, long and smooth. With continual training breathing will combine with movement, but should never be forced for this purpose. In each movement the whole framework of the body must be in use, the four limbs, trunk and head should move as one. One part moves, al the component parts move. This movement should be from the centre of gravity.

For the novice, the most important thing is to remember these points and grasp the principles. Each movement of the Form should be practised many times. It is not necessary to look for quick success. Benefits are progressive, persistent practice is the mode for a high level of achievement. In China, it is a common practise to train early morning and evening, repeating the Form many times. If time does not permit, it is recommended to practise at least once a day.

The actions of the feet should be light but firm and take an example from gentle movements of a cat while the legs should illustrate the principle of distinguishing substantial from insubstantial. Relaxation of the body and mind makes us ask what real relaxation is and what does in mean in Taijiquan and to the Chinese. To pay attention 100% to the movements and eliminate all extraneous thoughts will bring quietness to the mind and nervous system. Relaxation of the whole body implies conscious attention to all parts of the skeletal framework, joints, muscles, ligaments, tendons and internal organs. Relaxation also means opening and stretching of the joints and limbs. The overall benefits to the Taiji practitioner are a feeling of deep relaxation and heaviness. This form of relaxation dissolves rigidity and stiffness. The development can progress deeper over the years with training and closely resembles what can be observed with infants. Notice when a baby grasps your finger while remain relaxed. You can experience a feeling of great firmness in their grasp. So Taijiquan relaxation gives rise, or perhaps it would be more correct to say lowers the gravity, and induces relaxation, which in turn lays a foundation for vigorous action.

The spiralling arc like movements of Taijiquan should manifest from the legs and waist and conform to a principle found in nature. While a strong flat wind can be destructive, the spiral of a typhoon whirlwind wreaks havoc in its capacity to lift and uproot objects in its path. This is also seen in the undertow in tidal movements of the sea. The movements of Taijiquan should be initiated in the legs, controlled by the waist and expressed in the hands and fingers. All parts of the body should move in step, illustrating a balanced whole. It is the actions of the legs and waist which combine to form the basis of all Taijiquan actions.

Stationary Push Hand

Stationary push hands incorporates the four (proper) push hands method which includes ward-off, roll back, press, and into a two person exercise. This push hands method is conducted in a stationary position. Based upon which hand and foot is placed to the front, stationary push hands can be further divided into four postures. When the left hand and left foot is forward, this posture is termed left joining hand in direct step; when the left hand and right foot are forward, the posture is termed left joining hand in cross step; when the right hand and right foot are forward, this is termed right joining hand in direct step; and when the right hand and left foot are forward, this posture is termed right joining hand in cross step. In the process of training in stationary push hands, all four methods should be mutually performed and understood. The following example of stationary push hands will use the method of left joining hand with cross step.

1) Preparatory Posture

A (represents one person) and B (represents the other person) stand upright facing each other. Both step the right foot to the front and join their left hands together. The back of the hands face inward and are crossed at the wrists. Next, the right hands are placed on the others left elbow. When your hands are joined, the mind and body should be tranquil and your arms should be relaxed and soft. However, the arms still must maintain a point of ward-off energy and the intent internally locked.

2) A - Push; B - Ward-off

A bends the right leg to form a bow stance while B bends the left leg and sits back. At the same time, A's two palms spiral inward pushing towards B; B's left palm spirals slightly outward crossing the arm to ward-off the push. At the same time, B's upper body begins to turn to the left.

Push: The intent is to push down and/or to the front. However, push in Taiji either has the intent of leading and crossing or lowering and rising. If one only pushes in forward fashion, it would be easy for others to control, but if the waist and legs are used properly, the opponent will feel fatigued and confused. Push will destroy press. One can either use either palms or one to push in a forward direction. Push will be used to first dissolve the incoming pressing movement, followed by a forward pushing motion with the power of the waist. In actuality, this technique is a circular motion. The upper body should never lean forward.

Ward-off: Ward off and roll back destroys push. Ward-off is a method of protecting ones self. If there was no ward-off energy in push hands, then the body would be overtaken by the opponent. When an opponent pushes, do not meet head on, but change and lead the push away with ward-off energy; afterwards, perform roll back against the opponent. Ward-off energy carries with it an upward and forward motion. Many people say that Taijiquan mainly consists of ward-off energy. There is a saying which states that when one is performing Taijiquan, ward-off energy always exists in the movement. Ward-off energy should not be stiff or hard. It must be soft and flexible like an elastic band. The arms must be circular and full and the arm pits must be empty to maintain agility. Even though ward-off energy is in the arms, it is generated in the waist.

3) B - Roll Back; C – Press

B follows the push from A by turning the body to the left while sitting back onto the rear leg. The left wrist follows the ward-off motion allowing A's ward-off energy to leave B's center; thereby borrowing the energy from A. Both hands roll back towards the left rear. The right arm rolls back and spirals outward as the left arm rolls back and spirals inwards. The right hand of A leaves the elbow of B and moves toward the inside of A's own elbow.

A's left arm forms a left ward-off arm posture as B rolls back. This is considered a hidden press technique. Roll Back: Roll back dissolves the attack of push. Roll back will be used when ward-off energy is not sufficient to complete the task. As the opponent draws near, roll back is performed to lead the opponent to the rear or to the side of the body. Roll back must be light, soft, adhering, following, and must be perfectly timed. Actions that move too fast are easy to be lost and those that move too slow are easy to hit head on. Roll back uses the intent of "borrowing the opponent's strength to issue internal energy". Ward-off and roll back are mutually connected. One will first use ward-off and then roll back. In the method of roll back one must coordinate the motion of the waist and legs.

4) A - Press; B - Push

A follows the motion of B's roll back by forming a bow stance and crossing the left arm towards B's right arm. A's left hand moves up and inward. A's right palm is placed on the inside of A's own left elbow with the palm faces down at an angle while pressing toward B's chest. B follows A's press and turns the waist to the right. Both arms slightly spiral inward to change into push.

Press: Press destroys roll back. Press is one of push hands main movements. Press is produced after the opponent begins to perform roll back. Press should not be conducted too high nor too low. The energy of press is a forward and downward type. Press can be used most effectively when the energy is reversed at the last moment of execution. Beginners who are leaving four corners push hands find press relatively difficult to perform properly at first. Press uses the forearm to press on the opponent's body. One can also use the back of the palm to press forward.

5) B - Push; A - Ward-off

B follows A's press as the waist continues to turn to the right. The upper body turns until it is facing square with A. At the same time, the arms continue to spiral inward whereby the right hand connects to A's right hand. The left hand sinks down to near A's right elbow. Following, both hands slightly moves down as they push forward while the right leg bends to from a bow stance. A's press changes into ward-off as the right arm deflects B's push.

A's upper body turns to the right as the left hand moves from below over to B's right elbow while still maintaining contact with B. Perform ward-off and then roll back towards the right. B then places the left hand near the inside of B's own right elbow and presses forward. A turns while performing push as B wards off the push. Continue repeating ward-off, roll back, press, and push in a fluent continuous manner. The heart of each technique is based upon change. Without properly changing at the right instance, the motion will not be continuously connected. After many years of training, the student will understand this energy

Single Hand Techniques – The Starting Position

1. Stand facing each other, at a distance of about three feet or 1 meter 2. Both partners A & B each have their right foot forward and placed side by side. 3. Right hands are raised to chest height. Put your right arm in a gentle curve in front of the body. 4. Your arms touch each other on the outer edges of the wrist, back of wrist to back of wrist (lightly). 5. The left arm is raised with the forearm at about waist height - used to counterbalance the movement of the right arm. 6. Bend the knees slightly. 7. Keep the upper back straight and the head upright. 8. Feet should be firm on the floor and kept perfectly still. Note The Starting Position can be reversed with the left foot and the left hand forward. As a beginner it is best to practice with a partner of your own body weight and height.

Start a series of rocking motions circling back and forth, each person remaining outside the other. Attempt to break each others balance by pushing and yielding. Fend off an attack by yielding and redirect the force pass your body. This is achieved by turning the waist and hips (thus turning the upper body) and by shifting your body weight forward and backward. At your partner's slightest pressure yield to them, at their slightest retreat sticks to them. Each in turn tries to unbalance the other while yielding and offering no resistance to their partner's push. Yielding to every muscular force creates a sixth sense that helps to counter your partner's move before they make it. By constantly attacking and defending you become fine tuned to feel the timing and the state of balance of your partner.

Each push comes in at a different angle, direction and force. If you have to move (step) because your own balance is wrong then it is an advantage to your partner. Avoid being "Double Weighted" - weight on both feet at the same time. Any resistance to your partner results in you being pushed. The actions are circular, moving arms vertically and horizontally. Your body weight should shift from the front to the rear. Use your upper waist and upper torso in the action. Feet remain fixed and do not move. Palms should be glued to your partner like a shadow to its object or as an echo to its sound. The three main focal points are.

    1. One owns centre of balance.

    2. Your partner's centre of balance.

    3. The relationship between the two.

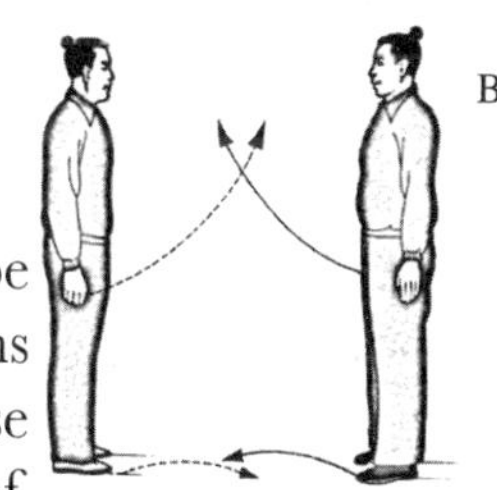

An expert offers no firm surface to be pushed. When you are off balance it means that your centre of gravity is outside the base made by your feet. The maximum point of your partner's reach usually means that they are almost completely off balance. Balance ultimately rests on your feet. If you are pushed from the rear you are usually able to grip the surface with the toes; if you are pushed from the front this is not possible.

Nine Steps for Single Hand Techniques

1. A turns over his right hand, using palm to push B's wrist; while at the same time A bends his right knee, shifting his weight forward a little and tries to reach the right-side of B's chest with his right hand. 2. B does not resist A's pressure and folds his arm toward his chest; while at the same time bends his left knee and shifts his weight back a little, turning his torso to the right and diverts A's hand away from the his chest with his right palm. 3. B turns over his right hand, using his palm to push A's wrist and tries to reach the right side of A's chest. 4. A does not resist B's pressure and bends his left knee, shifting his weight backward and turns his torso to his right, using his right palm to ward off B's right hand. 5. Both A & B return to starting position. A turns his right hand over, using his palm to B's wrist forward and up and tries to reach for B's face; while at the same time bends his right knee and shifts his weight forward a little. B does not resist A's force and takes advantage of the situation by lifting his arm by

bending his left knee slightly, shifting his body weight back a little and turning his torso to the right and diverts A's hand away to the right of his head. 6. B slowly presses his right down and forward and tries to reach for A's right ribs. 7. A does not resist B's force and withdraws his right arm; while at the same time bends his left knee, shifting his weight back a little, turning his torso to the right and diverts B's hand away to the right of his body. 8. A reaches for B's face with his right hand, while B turns to his right to divert A's hand away to the right of his head. 9. B takes advantage of A's movements by reaching for A's face. A counters by bending his left leg a little, turning his body to the right to neutralize B's force, and continues to push down and forward with his palm and reaches for B's right ribs. Repeat this cycle as many times as possible until you know it.

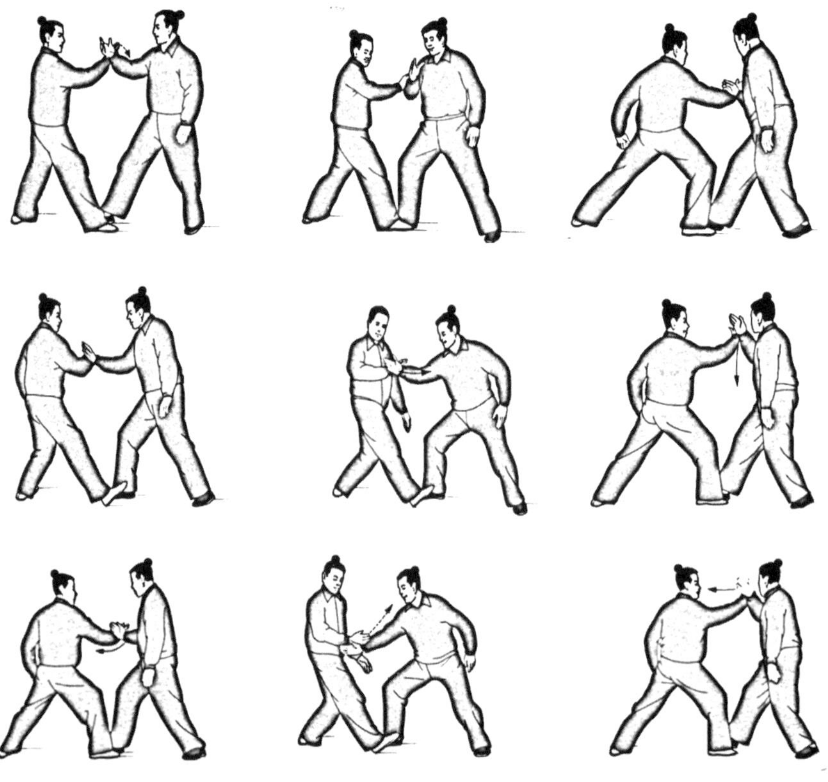

Two Handed Pushing Hand Techniques

After some experience of working single handed Pushing Hands, those interested are encouraged to progress onto double handed contact. The starting position is identical to the single handed stance but both hands will now be used. Moving and stepping is also introduced at this stage. Both hands may touch simultaneously. When changing over from one hand to the other it is important that two-hand contact is made before the changeover takes place. Contact with your partner must always be maintained with at least one hand.

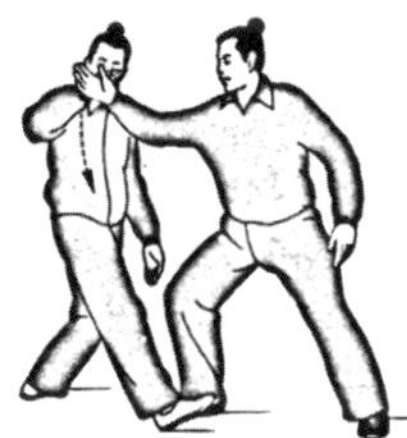
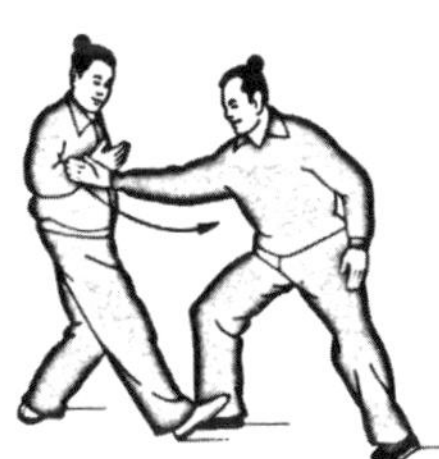

Five Steps For Two-Hand Techniques

1. Come into starting position as in single handed contact. 2. A turns over his right hand so that his palm is touching B's right wrist and forces B to withdraw to his right arm toward his in a forward and downward move; while at the same time A moves his left hand forward in the same direction from B's elbow. 3. B accepts A's forward force with his arm and retreats with his left hand resting on A's right elbow. B bends his left leg slightly,

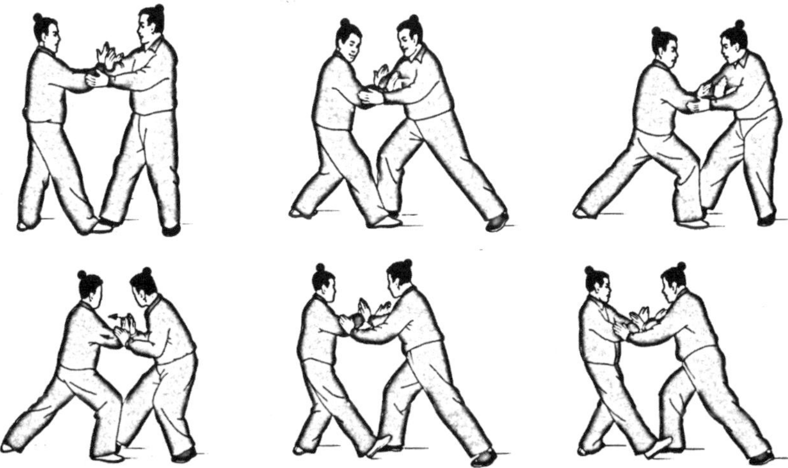

shifting his weight backward, turning his torso to the right and use his right arm to divert A's push to the right, thus ending A's force. 4. B turns over his right hand so that his palms touches A's right wrist; while at the same time pushes both palms forward and downward forcing A to withdraw his right arm toward his chest; while at the same time moves his left hand forward in the same direction from A's elbow. 6. A accepts B's forward force with his arm and retreats with his left hand resting on B's right elbow. A bends his left leg slightly, shifting his weight backward, turning his torso to the right and use his right arm to divert B's push to the right, thus ending B's force. Repeat this cycle as many times until you know it.

Pushing Hands on Fixed Feet

1. Stand facing each other, at a distance of about three feet or 1 meter 2. Both partners A & B each have their right foot forward and placed side by side. 3. Raise your right hand with your left elbow bent and backs of the hands lightly touching each other. Do not press too hard or yield too much to each other. 4. A retreats by turning his body to the right and then withdrawing his right arm. A turning his right hand over and touching B's right wrist: while at the same time gently holds B's right elbow with his left hand and takes advantage of B's forward force bends his left knee and turns his waist to the right, with his hands in a pull-back movement, inviting B's arm in. 5-6. B follows A's withdrawing movement, bending his right knee and shifting his body weight forward; while at the same time moves his left hand inside his right forearm and presses it toward A's chest and tries to force A to abandon his effort. Next A takes advantage of B's forward force and bends his left leg; while pulling his chest in and turning his waist to the left and press B'[s right arm down and to the left with his both hands, thereby neutralizing B's pressing force. 7. A moves his right hand to B's left elbow and his left hand to B's left wrist and pushes forward with his palms. 8-9. B accepts A's push with his left arm and pulls his right hand out to hit A's left elbow: while at the same time bends his left leg, shifting his body weight backward and turns his body slightly to his left, defending

120

against A's force with his left arm and deflects A's arm upward with both hands, and with a pulling out movement lures A's arm in. 10. A takes immediate advantage of B's move and with his right hand supporting inside of his left elbow press firmly forward to B's chest. 11. B accepts A's forward force and bends his left leg, pulling his chest in and moving his hands to A's right elbow. 12. B shifts his body weigh forward and pushes A's right arm away to the right. 13. A raises his right hand to ward off B's push and at the same time moves his left hand to hold B's right elbow and turns his body to the right. 14. B presses his right arm forward to A's chest. A instead of resisting B, holds B's left wrist with his left hand and pushes B's left elbow gently with his right hand; while turning his body to the left and diverts B's pressure. 15. B with his left leg bent takes advantage of the situation by pressing his left arm forward. 16. When A responds by pushing forward with both his hands B moves his left hand from underneath A's hands to hold A's right elbow and shifts his body weight backward, enticing A in. At this point A pushes forward. Repeat this cycle as many times until you know it, remembering to move backward and forward, without moving feet.

Pushing Hands on Feet Moving

Pushing hands on moving feet It is said, to "Lure the opponent's advance into emptiness; harmonize with him, then issue power. Adhere, join, stick to and follow the opponent, without letting go or resisting," (that is, follow the opponent on both the vertical and horizontal planes) while at the same time be aware of the position of the feet as the go forward and backward.

As the feet move follow the opponent's incoming posture and lead him into emptiness. As I lead him in, I issue my own attack. The word "lead" actually has two meanings. The first is to accord with the opponent's posture and draw him further in order to take advantage [of his momentum]. The second is to feign weakness, causing him to rush in brashly. Entice the opponent with an 'empty basket'; then just make one turn." Enticing with an empty basket is the same as "Lure the opponent's advance into emptiness." "Turning" means striking the opponent.

1. Stand facing each other, at a distance of about three feet or 1 meter 2. A puts his left foot forward and B puts his right foot forward on the outside of A's left foot. 3. Both raise their left hands with elbows bent and backs of their hands touching each other. Each person's right hand should touch the other's left elbow. 4. A presses forward with his left arm and rest his right hand on the inside of B's elbow; while B pushes A's arm down with both his hands. 5. B places his right foot on the inside of A's left foot and pushes A's arm with both hands. 6. A steps back with his left foot, and takes hold of B's right hand and hits B's right elbow with his left hand. B benefits from A's retreat and brings his left foot forward and lands it just outside of A's right foot and gets ready to press forward with his right arm. 7. A steps back with his right foot; while at the same time directs B's arm to the right with both his hands. Following A's withdrawal, B brings his right foot forward again and places it just inside A's left foot with his right knee bent and his arm pressing forward. 8. A bends his right knee slightly, shifting his body weight backward and pushes at B's arms with his hands. 9. A take advantage of B pressing forward and turns his waist slightly to the left, lifting his left foot and lands it on the inside of B's right foot and pushes forward with both his hands. 10. B steps back with his right foot and at the same time moves his right hand around and takes hold of A's elbow and move backs. A takes advantage of B's move and brings his right foot forward landing it just outside B's left foot. 11. B retreats with his left foot; while at the same time A follows with his left foot and places it just inside B's right foot, and presses forward again with his left arm. B pushes A's arm downward with both his hands and returns to step 4. Repeat this cycle as many times until you know it, remembering to move backward and forward, moving backward and forward etc.

Advance Three Steps & Retreat Three Steps

No matter whether one practices the form or push-hands, one should avoid straight advance or straight retreat. The Explanation of Practice says, "Advancing and retreating require turning the body and changing the steps." The meaning is that one must not linearly advance or linearly retreat. For instance, in the advancing motion of you must look to the left and right. Or in the retreating motion of you must similarly turn and step towards the left and right. All the advancing and retreating movements are like this. Because turning and changing allow you to use the retreat as an advance, it is not a true retreat. A true retreat would mean defeat. Therefore the ancient boxing treatises say, "Advancing is advancing. Retreating is also advancing,"

Finally, when each person advances and retreats, A advances a step by warding-off, another step with elbow, a further step with press and a finally, a close step with shoulder-stroke. B rolls-back with three retreating steps. Then he turns his body, stepping behind me. This last step embraces the movements of pull-down, split and push. Because there are three retreating steps utilizing roll-back, the exercise is called "big roll-back". No matter what push-hands method you practice, it is most important not to neglect the principles and not to use force in attack and defense. Furthermore, you should have absolutely no thought of win or loss.

Starting Position

A & B both half turn to your left and step forward with your right foot and raise your right hands, elbows bent and backs of your hands lightly touching each other; do not press or retreat from each other too much. 1 – 3. A presses forward with his left arm, aiming for B's chest, while support himself with the inside of this left elbow and his right hand and right leg bent. B retreats and pushes at A's arm with both hands: while at the same time B lifts his right foot and steps forward and A lifts his left foot and steps backward. B with his right hand takes hold of A's right hand causes A's right arm to fold and hits A's right elbow with his left hand. 4-5. B advances again with his left foot and A retreats with his right foot. A raises his right hand to ward off B's push and at the same moves his left hand to hold B's right elbow and turns his body to his right. B continues to advance with his right foot and A continues to retreat with his left foot. B presses forward with his left arm, aiming at A's chest, while supporting the inside of his left elbow with his right hand. A pushes at B's arm with both his hands; while at the same time retreating backwards. 6-10 Repeat steps 1-5, A starts by stepping forward with his right foot and B starts by stepping backward with his left foot. Repeat this cycle as many times until you know it, remembering to move backward and forward, moving backward and forward etc.

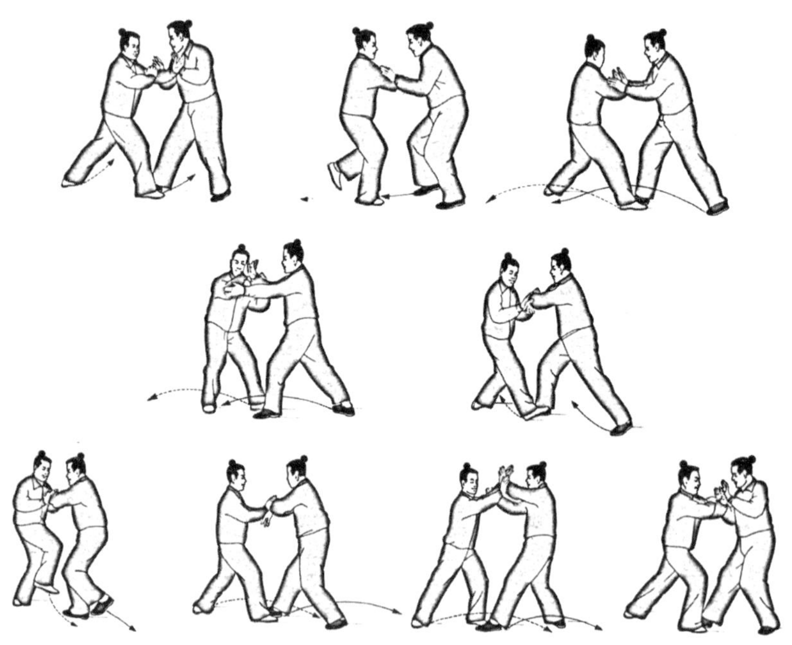

DA-LU

Da-Lu is to pull back. As an oncoming force is detected A steps slightly to the side and backwards, blocking upward using our most potent blocking method.. We then take a further step with our other foot diagonally and use pull back as our opponent takes a further step to counter this directive pull. Our opponent B then takes another side step to in between our two legs and barges in with shoulder to counter the pull and in keeping with the Taiji principle of going with the force and not against it. This exercise continues with both A & B stepping in turn into each corner of an imaginary square.

124

Da-Lu can become quite energetic with both partners actually lifting off the ground with the centrifugal force generated by this pushing hands method. Da-Lu should only be used however when there is something wrong with our foundation postures. It is a way of getting out of trouble when we are attacked at a weak point. For instance, if you have not developed a good enough grounding/centre, then your partner will be able to grab your arm and pull you to the side and forward. Use Da-Lu to counter this. However, if your grounding was good enough then your partner should not have been able to pull you forward in the first place. So Da-Lu is a technique we use when our basic techniques are not up to scratch. It should be remembered that Da-Lu still doesn't teach us how to defend ourselves.

1. A& B turn to their left and put their right foot forward and raise the right hand, elbow bent and the back of the hands lightly touching each other. 2 A turns over his right hand, holding B's right wrist gently and rests his left hand on B's right elbow, while at the same A rotates on the ball of his left foot, half turning to his right, bringing his right foot back and starts pulling back. B moves his left foot next to his right foot and shifts his body weight forward. 3 A turns his body to his right and steps back with his right foot; while at the same time keeps pulling back B's arm with his both arms, forcing B to step forward with his left foot. 4. Following A's pulling, B brings his right forward, just inside A's left foot and shifts his weight onto his right leg; while at the same holds the inside of his right arm with his left hand and leans shoulders lightly against A's chest. 5-6. A takes advantage of B's move, and catches B's right arm with his left arm and elbow and turns his body slightly to the right so as to defuse B's forward force. A then pulls his chest in, turning his waist to the left and shifts his weight to the right leg; while at the same starts to push forward instead of pulling back by putting his left hand on B's left hand and right hand on B's left elbow and brings his left foot forward so that it lands on inside of B's left foot. 7. B accepts A's forward push and stops A's hand with his left forearm and moves his right arm around to hold A's left elbow; while at the same time B pulls right foot back, turning his body slightly to the left and starts to pull. As B moves, A bends his left leg and shifts his body weight forward.

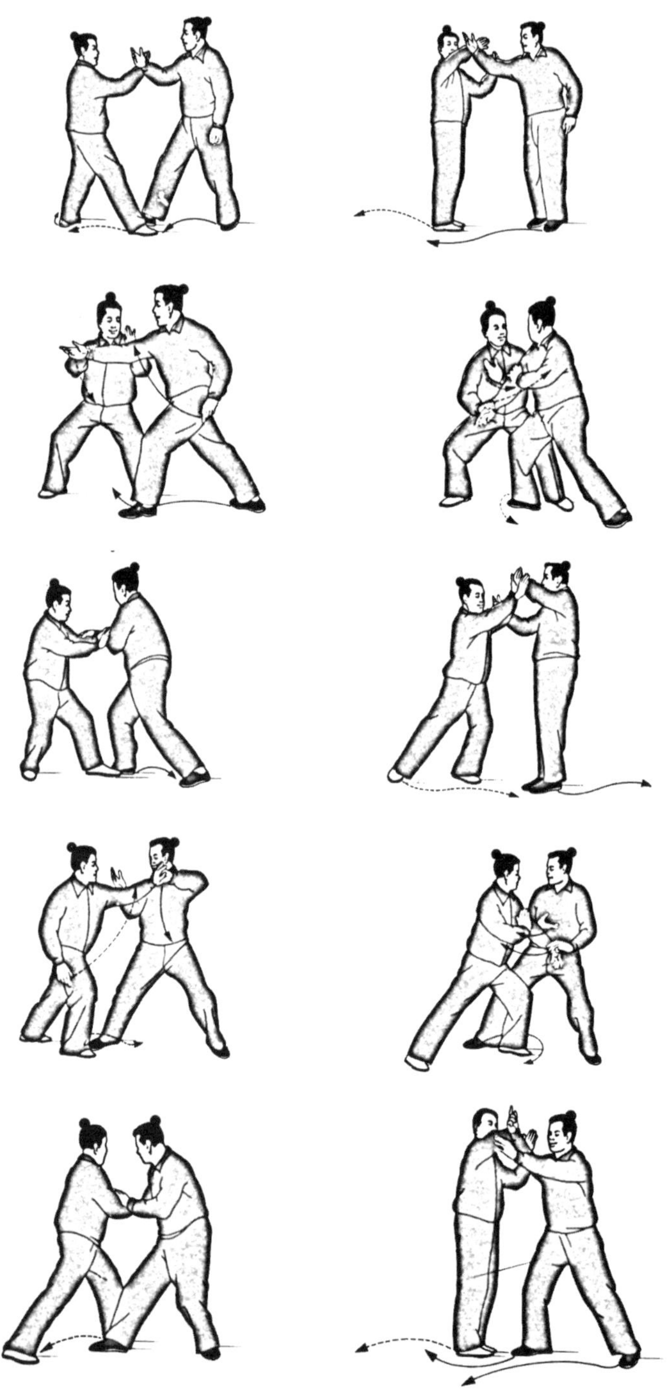

8. B turns his body to the left, and steps back with his left foot, bending his knee; while at the same time continues to pull A's left wrist with his left hand and his left elbow with his right hand. A follows by taking a long step forward with his right foot and shifting his weight onto his right leg; while A follows with his foot, putting it on the outside of B's right foot and shifting his weight forward. At the same time with his right hand pressing inside his left arm, leans his shoulder toward B's chest. Repeat this cycle as many times until you know it, remembering that A & B both advance and retreat – if B advances with his right foot and pushes forward while A retreats with his left foot and pulls back.

Changing Hands Method

1. B steps forward with his left foot and leans his right arm and shoulder against A's chest; while B takes another step forward with his right foot and A steps back with his right foot. A, while stepping back, turns his body to the right and receives and defuses B's forward force with his left arm and at the same time quickly raises his right hand as though about to hit B's face. 2. B raises his right arm to ward off A's hand and steps back with his right foot; while at the same time B turns his body to the right, keeping his feet together, and pulls A to the right by holding A's right wrist with his right hand and right elbow with his left hand. 3. A follows with his right foot, shifting his weight forward and turns to his left. 4. B keeps turning to the right, stepping back with his right foot and continues to pull A. A brought in by B's pulling movement, steps forward with his left foot, and makes a complete right turn and puts his right foot on the inside of B's left foot; while at the same time pushes inside the right arm with his hand and leans forward against B's chest. 5-8. A steps forward and leans his left arm and shoulder against B's chest. B turns his body to the left, using his right arm to receive and neutralize A's onward force. At the same time raises his left hand quickly as though about to hit A's face. A uses his left hand to pull B's left arm to the left. B follows with his left arm and presses it against A's chest. Repeat this cycle as many times until you know it, remembering to move backward and forward, moving backward and forward etc.

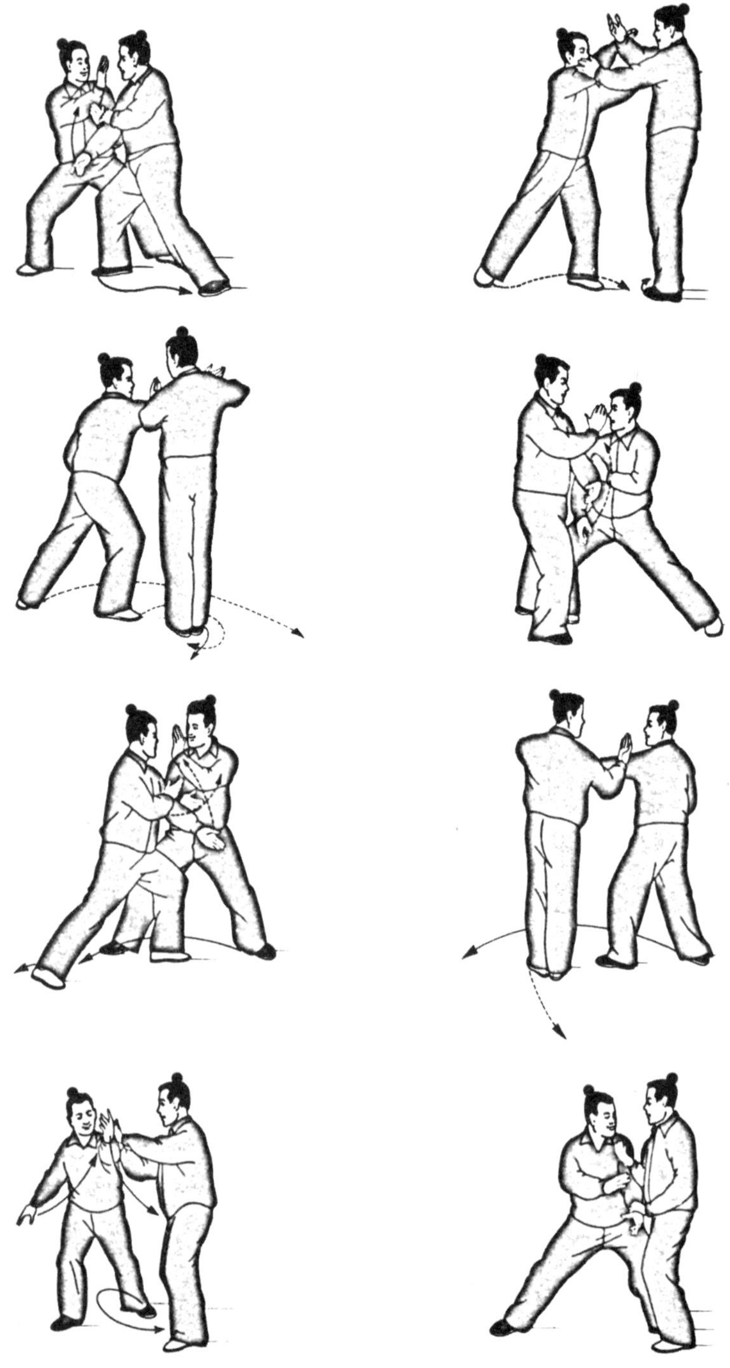

Self Healing

Self-Healing shows you how to be aware of your thoughts and your feelings, how to listen to your body, and understand how it works and how it communicates with you. Thoughts form a big part of self-healing.

There is a self-healing aspect which is part of every person's body, mind and spirit. In most cultures the traditional healing system is based on enhancing and supporting this inborn healing energy. For some reason knowledge of how to enhance our automatic healing impulse has been lost in the Western world until very recently. For several hundred years we have believed that the disease comes from outside and attacks the individual who is a helpless victim. Many disorders including heart disease, diabetes, stroke and cancer have been found to be largely preventable. We are now realizing that even though the disease may come from the outside, as in a virus, the internal healing mechanism of the

immune system is the most important healer. The best and most profound medicine is already in us. We must learn and apply methods to activate the medicine within and its ability to heal us.

Self-health responsibility, more than any other possible option, is the solution to our healing. Evidence for the truth of this fact is coming at us from everywhere. Research has shown that diet, exercise and stress management are powerful tools for maintaining health. However, in the Western world we have little tradition that is well tried in support of self-health actions. Diets change every day. Jogging was thought to be a perfect system but now has been found to be less beneficial than simple walking. Aerobics sold a great deal of equipment but was found to be detrimental to many people. Now low impact aerobics is the latest approach.

The Qigong of China is a system of self-applied health enhancement which is easy to learn and simple to apply. Self-care is one of the most important features of the Asian traditional systems of medicine. These ancient philosophical and medical theories encourage, and, in fact, demand action and responsibility on the part of the person who is seeking to maintain or enhance health.

The self-application of health enhancement methods is particularly remarkable because of the broad array of real health benefits that are triggered. These practices modify and accelerate the body's own self-regulating physiological and bioenergetics mechanisms. They have a very practical application for healing diseases as well as supporting health maintenance, endurance and longevity. In addition, the very same practices, refined, deepened, and perfected, link to a whole realm of more metaphysical practices focused toward spiritual growth.

In the modern Western world the prevailing medical system is tragically lacking in strategies that a person or patient can implement themselves to support their own healing process. Aside from being patient and compliant to the physician's orders there has generally been little that the patient could do. The self-applied health enhancement methods that spring from the Asian traditions are tried and true techniques refined over thousands of years that are ready to be used now.

A rapidly expanding health care revolution in the areas of patient responsibility and patient action is necessary immediately to meet the urgent need for solutions to the crisis in medical costs and the crisis in quality of care. These health enhancement practices lend themselves completely and readily to the critical need for patient applied self-care which complements any clinical strategy whether it be as conservative as acupuncture or as radical as surgery.

Beginning level of self-applied health practices are:

Relaxation Techniques
Breath Activities
Eye Movement
Massages of the Body
Body Soaks

These are easy to learn, easy to apply, require no special knowledge or training and can be practiced by the whole family and all people (sick or well) daily with very little impact on time or energy. In fact, they actually give the individual, both time and energy. Time is gained because there is less fatigue and forgetfulness, and energy is gained because the function of the organs and glands is enhanced and regenerated. Every minute spent applying these methods is returned to the practitioner in a need for less sleep. Every unit of energy spent brings forth an internal ability to generate an even greater amount of energy.

The preliminary methods of Qigong can be learned and practiced as individual techniques. However, integrated into a singular practice they become even more powerful. This integration of relation techniques, breathing activities, cyc movement, massages of the body and body soaks, saves on time which is so precious to most people in Western culture. Traditions of this type of practice from both China have integrated the five preliminary methods for thousands of years into systems that are highly refined. The preliminary methods are profound in effect and yet extremely simple to learn and apply. Especially in the Chinese arts of Tai Chi and Qigong, the methods are merged into a singular practice which is sometimes called moving meditation or meditation in motion. In China, literally millions of people practice these methods daily. Children in schools, industrial workers in factories, elders in the parks and patients in hospitals all apply the preliminary methods faithfully on a daily basis.

Relaxation Techniques

Strengthening and Relaxing Body Remedies

1. Exercise The Neck

Many people suffer from neck stiffness arid soreness, and its no wonder your neck has the difficult burden of carrying your bead around, and it never gets a break except when you lay down. This neck push can be done sitting or standing and helps strengthen your neck muscles, which in turn will help alleviate some of the discomfort.

Breathe in; keeping your head upright, hold the palm of one hand against your forehead, and press your head forward, resisting with your palm. Hold for 10 to 15 seconds. Breathe out; now clasp your hands behind your head, and press your head backward, resisting with your hands. Hold for 10 to 15 seconds. Breathe in; now hold your right hand against the side of your head, and press your head to the right, resisting with your hand. Again, hold for 10 to 15 seconds. Then repeat on left side.

Relax and Roll Stress and anxiety often lead to an aching neck. Poor posture also plays a role. This stretch relieves tension in your neck and surrounding muscles. Relax your shoulders and let your head roll forward, chin to chest. Slowly rotate your head in a circle without straining your neck. Repeat five times.

Relax. Then rotate in the opposite direction and repeat five times. Try not to raise your shoulders as you do this exercise.

2. Exercise the Shoulders

This stretch is best done in a standing position. It is great not only for your shoulders, but also your triceps (backs of your arms). Do several times a day, or whenever your shoulders and upper body are feeling tight. Breathe in; standing upright, push both arms straight back with your palms facing down and hold for five seconds. Breathe out; bend in arms at the elbow (like a hinge), fingers pointing straight ahead, and hold for five seconds. Repeat five to 10 times.

Swinging your arms like you are hitting the ground

Try for maximum stretch to relieve the tension in your shoulders and elbows that develops as you work at your keyboard all day. Breathe in; from a standing position, clasp your hands and hold them close to your right shoulder, as though resting an ax there. Gently swing your arms by straightening your elbows and moving your hands toward your left thigh. Breathe out; raise your clasped hands to your left shoulder, and swing your arms toward your right thigh. Repeat on both sides seven or eight times.

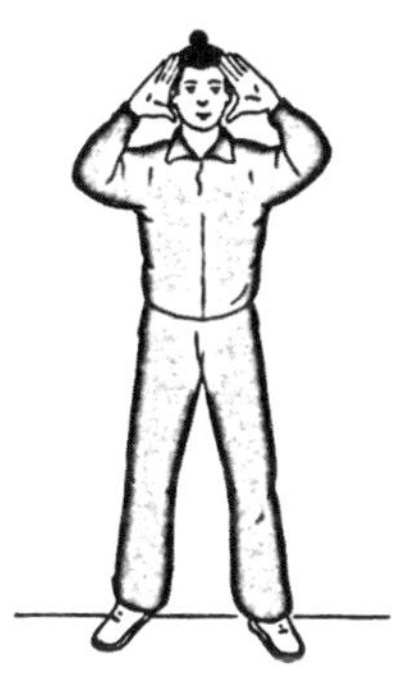 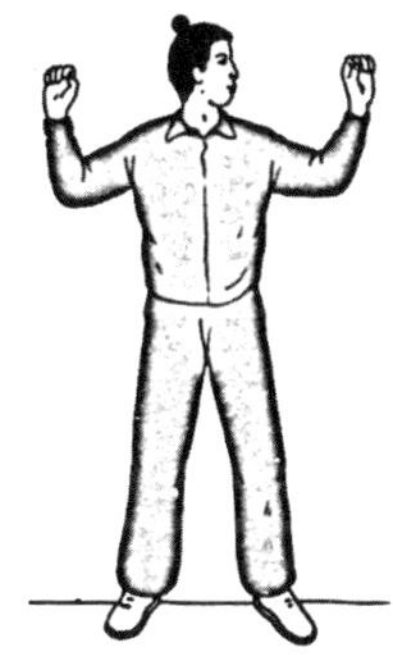

Shoulder Movements

Your shoulders are the link between the three most common sites of stress-related pain - your head, neck and back. Increasing flexibility in your shoulders will also help with back and neck relaxation. Breathe in; sitting erect in a chair. Raise your arms so that elbows are flared in an outward position and hands are at shoulder level in front of your body. Breathe out; keep hands at shoulder level and push your elbows as high as you can, isolating the pressure on your shoulders. Repeat 10 to 15 times. Perform the first few slowly and smoothly, the next few faster and more intense, and the last couple slow and smooth.

Shake your shoulders

Loosen up your shoulders, chest and back by shaking your shoulders. It takes only a minute and releases a lot of tension in your upper body. It can be done from either a sitting or standing position. Breathe in; place your fingertips on your shoulders, elbows pointing out to the sides. Pull your elbows back as far as you can. Breathe out; push your elbows forward and try to touch them together. Breathe in; keeping your fingertips on your shoulders, lift your elbows up and then push them down to your sides, as if you're trying to fly. Repeat this cycle 10 times.

Shoulder Roll

Your shoulders are one of the most flexible joints in your body, when they are functioning smoothly. Does this shoulder roll at least three times a day to relax your shoulders? You may do this one shoulder at a time, or both together.

Breathe in; sit or stand tall. Lift your shoulders as high as you can. Breathe out; bring them forward. Push them down. Breathe in; pull your shoulders back. Breathe out; returning to starting position. Repeat in the opposite direction. Repeat the following cycle five times.

3. Exercising the Arms

Stretch Your Arms High to the Sky

This stretch relieves tension in your arms, sides and waist. It feels great when done slowly and smoothly, so take your time and don't rush it. Perform the stretch first thing in the morning and periodically throughout the day.

Stretch your arms up, one at a time, as high as you can, as if reaching for the sky. Breathe in; come into a standing position with your legs straight feet together. Breathe out; lift your right arm above your head with your right hand pointing to the sky; while at the same time pulling your left arm down with your left hand pointing downward. Breathe in; come back into standing position. Breathe out; lift your left arm above your head with your left hand pointing to the sky; while at the same time pulling your right arm down with you're your left hand pointing downward. Breathe in; come back into standing position. Repeat theis cycle 10 times.

Push-ups

These stand-up push-ups are easier than the military kind. Nevertheless, they build up strength in the arms and shoulders and doing them feels great when you are stiff from sitting all day. All you need is a wall to lean on, so stand up and push. Stand facing a wall, with your fleet apart and about 12 inches from the wall. Rest your palms on the wall at about shoulder height. Bend your elbows and lean toward the wall as far as possible without touching your forearms to the wall. Keep your legs and back straight. Push yourself back to starting position. The farther from the wall you stand, the greater the shoulder effort needed to push back. Gradually increase your distance as you become stronger, but don't exceed two feet.

4. Exercising the Hands and Wrists

Reach Out and Touch Your Fingers

This simple hand exercise will help to increase the mobility of your fingers. It's easily done at your desk several times a day. Do each hand individually. Touch the tip of your thumb to the tip of each finger in turn, making the circle as round as you can. Straighten your fingers in between touching each finger.

5. Exercising the Buttocks

Tighten your buttocks

Whether you sit all day or not, buttocks are an area of the body that we often neglect until we notice the area increasing in size! This exercise can be done while sitting in a chair or lying on your back with your knees bent. Do it several times a day to tighten those buttocks. Tighten and squeeze your buttocks, hold five to ten seconds, and release. Repeat six to eight times. Really concentrate on the "squeeze" for maximum results.

6. Exercising the Back and Upper Body

Twisting the Upper Torso

Breathe in; come to a standing position with legs shoulder-width apart, arms to your side. Breathe out; stretching both arms above your head with palms facing each other. Breathe in; Lower your arms and place them on your waist thumbs in front. Breathe out; twist your body toward the left with your eyes following the movement. Keep your chin as close to your shoulders. Breathe in; come back to the center. Breathe out; twist your body toward the right with your eyes following the movement. Keep your chin as close to your shoulders. Breathe in; come back to the center. Repeat this cycle 4 times.

Twisting your upper body

This torso twist stretch for the entire upper body can be done sitting right in your chair at the office or at home. Perform it several times a day, whenever you get that "tense" feeling in your body. Sit erect in a stationary chair with both feet flat on the floor. Look straight ahead. Slowly tilt your torso to the right as you reach around behind yourself with your right hand. Grasp the top right corner of your chair with your right hand. Complete the stretch by moving your left hand as close as possible to your right hand. Stretch as far as you can and hold it for 15 seconds. Repeat four to six times, twisting left and right, aiming to turn the body a little farther each time.

Twisting the Body and Looking Backward

This can be done standing done as many times as possible to relieve pain and stiffness in neck, shoulders, waist and legs. Breathe in; come into a standing position with legs shoulder-width apart, arms to your side. Breathe out; twist your body to the left with your right leg straight and left leg bent, look over your left shoulder; while at the same time stretch your right arm up, palm facing out, keep your right arm and leg in a straight line. Breathe in; return to a standing position with legs shoulder-width apart, arms to your side. Breathe out; twist your body to the right

with your left leg straight and your right leg bent, look over to
your right, while at the same time stretch your left arm up, palm
facing out, keep your left arm and leg in a straight line. Breathe
in; return to a standing position with legs shoulder-width apart,
arms to your side. Repeat this cycle 4 times.

Tummy Twist

Performing this range of motion exercise several times a day
will help prevent that tight, uncomfortable feeling in the trunk of
your body that comes from sitting all day. Stand with your feet
shoulder width apart. Hold your bent elbows down at your sides
with fists up. Lean slightly forward and twist side to side with your
elbows leading the movement. Repeat for 30 to 45 seconds.

Reach and Stretch

This stretch is good for your arms and body trunk. Done slowly,
it also serves as a great relaxation technique. Try very hard not
to bend forward as you lean-to the right or left. Stand with your
feet spread shoulder width apart. Raise one arm, then bend over
sideways reaching over your head, until your arm is parallel to
the floor (or as far as you can). Hold for five to 10 seconds. Repeat
with the other arm the same stretch.

Stretching Behind

This is a good way to "open-up" the chest muscles after you have
been sitting, leaning forward all day at your desk. Interlace your
fingers behind your back, palms facing in. Raise and straighten
your arms, squeezing your shoulder blades together and "opening
up" your chest. Fold for five to ten seconds. Repeat five to ten
times.

7. Exercising the Legs

Sitting in Mid-Air

Strengthen your weary, neglected legs as you have a "seat." If you have a wall and two to four minutes, try this exercise once a day. You'll definitely feel the results! Stand with your back against a wall and feet apart and about 16 inches from the wall. Lower yourself into a seated position, keeping feet flat on the floor, and hold for 15 to 30 seconds. Return to standing and relax for 30 seconds. Repeat three times. Do not bend your knees beyond a 90-degree angle.

Stretch legs

Weak or tight leg muscles often lead to back problems, which can make sitting for long periods uncomfortable. Legs are the foundation of good posture, and keeping them properly stretched prevents misalignment in the upper body.

Stand with your feet comfortably apart, your toes turned slightly outward. Hold the back of a chair if you need support. Keep your back straight and slowly bend your knees over your toes. (Its important not to extend your knees beyond your toes in order to avoid stress on the knees.) Straighten, by pushing up through your feet.

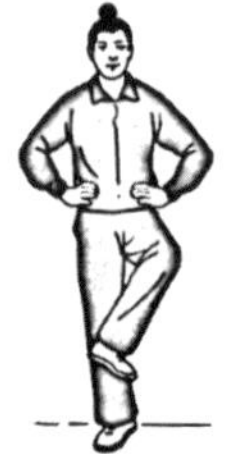 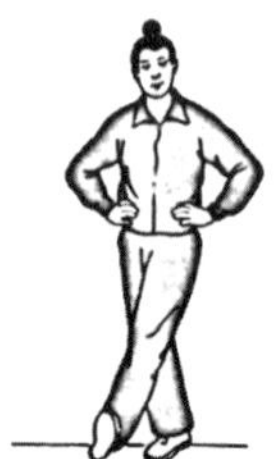

8. Exercising the Knees

Rotating Your Knees

Bend forward and place your hands on your knees. Rotate your knees clockwise four times and then counter clockwise 4 times. Repeat this cycle 4 times.

Squatting

Breathe in; come to a standing position. Breathe out; and bend forward and place your hands on your knees. Breathe out and squat with your hands on your knees. Breathe in; and place your hands on top of your feet and straighten your legs. Breathe out and come back in standing position. Repeat this cycle 4 times.

Bending and Stretching

Breathe in: standing with your legs apart, shoulder-width apart. Breathe out; bend forward, placing your right hand on your left knee while keeping your legs straight. Breathe in; bending your knees slightly, lift your left hand above your head, palm up, and keep your eyes on the back of your hands. Breathe out; straightening your legs and place your left hand on your right knee. Breathe in; and return to standing position with shoulder-width apart. Repeat this cycle in the opposite direction. Once you complete both directions repeat the full cycle 4 times.

Bending Knee to Chest

Breathe in; come into a standing position with legs straight feet together. Breathe out; step forward with your left foot and keeping your right heel off the ground, shift your body weight onto the left leg; while at the same time lift your arms above your head with your palms facing each other, keeping your head back and chest high. Breathe in; raising your right knee and drop your arms to your side. Clasp your hands around your right knee pressing tightly toward your chest while keeping your left leg straight. Breathe out; return to standing position. Breathe in; step forward with your right foot and keeping your left heel off the ground, shift your body weight onto the right leg; while at the same time lift your arms above your head with your palms facing each other, keeping your head back and chest high. Breathe out; raising your left knee and drop your arms to your side. Clasp your hands around your left knee pressing tightly toward your chest while keeping your left leg straight. Breathe in; return to standing position. Repeat the following cycle 4 times.

Sitting In a Chair

Breathe in; come into a standing position with legs shoulder-width apart, arms to your side. Breathe out; bend your knees and imagine your are sitting in a chair, while at the same time bring your arms straight in front of you at chest level and turn your arms in, open your fists and thrust open your palms forward with the middle fingers touching each other. Breathe in; and return to standing position with legs shoulder-width apart, arms to your side. Repeat this 4 times.

9. Exercising the Hamstrings

Stretch the Hamstrings

When you sit throughout the day, those leg muscles can become tight if you don't stretch them periodically. This exercise will get you out of your chair and help increase the flexibility in your hamstrings. Do twice a day if possible.

From a standing position, extend one leg out in front of your other leg about 10 inches, lifting your toes and digging your heel into the ground. Bend the back leg slightly, and put both hands on the thigh of your back leg to support your weight. You should feel the stretch in the back of your front leg. Hold for 10 to 15 seconds. Now push the toes of the front leg down to the floor and hold for another 10 to 15 seconds. Repeat on the other side.

Hamstring Curls

When you sit a lot during the day, its a good idea to take a break every couple of hours to do this exercise. It will strengthen the hamstrings (backs of legs above knees) - follow with a hamstring stretch for optimal results. Stand and hold on to something stable for support, such as a file cabinet or bookshelf. Slowly lift one heel toward your buttocks, then lower. The knee of the supporting leg should be slightly bent during the exercise, not locked. Repeat 12 to 15 times on each side. At home try using ankle weights for added resistance.

Balancing Stretch

This is the best stretch for the quadriceps muscles - the large group of muscles in the fronts of your legs above the knees. You may find it difficult to do at first, but it will get easier if you do it daily and your flexibility increases. Stand at the side of a chair with your left hand holding the chair for balance. Grab your right foot with your right hand (or grab your pant leg if you cannot reach your foot). Using your hand, pull your foot toward your buttocks and hold for 10 to 15 seconds. Your knee should be pointing downward, not out to the side. Repeat two to three times with each leg. To work on improving your balance, try removing your hand from the chair, little by little, as you hold the stretch.

Hamstring Hug

This is a good stretch for your lower body that you can do while sitting. Not only does it stretch your hamstrings - the group of muscles in the backs of your legs and above the knees, but you will also feel it working your quadriceps in the fronts of your legs. Sit back and place your hands under your right thigh. Pull knee toward chest then extend the leg straight in front of you as far as you can. Repeat with your other leg the same stretch. Do three to five times with each leg.

10. Exercising the Feet and Ankles

The following are two exercises; one for the office and one for home. A big part of being able to do embellishments well is having strong, flexible and stable feet and ankles. After all, you will often find yourself standing on one leg, balancing with your weight over the ball of your foot, and you also need to take controlled, strong steps backwards. If your feet are out of alignment, the rest of your body will be too.

Each foot alone contains 26 bones, 33 muscles, 31 joints and over 100 ligaments (!), so don't dance as though they were just stumps at the end of your legs. Use every muscle each time you step.

Here are a few exercises that will build foot strength and will also help you articulate through your feet.

Point and Flex at the Office

This exercise can be done under your desk at work all day long: Sit in a chair and take off your shoes. Raise your legs off the floor so they are straight out in front of you. (If you can't get them straight that's fine, just raise them as much as you are able.) Point both your feet strongly from the ankles. It is like you are trying to get your toes to curl down to touch the bottom of your heel as the arch of your foot rounds upwards. Hold this position for 2 minutes.

Now, maintain this foot position in the ankle and arch, but isolate just your toes and flex them back like you are trying to touch them to the front of your ankle. Hold this position for 2 minutes.

Now, flex both feet, bending them towards you at the ankle as if you were trying to get the top of the arches and the toes to fold up against your shins. Hold this position for 2 minutes.

Circle the feet clockwise from the ankles, feeling the feet, roll through a point, then to the side, then a flex, and around to the remaining side. Make 10 full, slow circles, and then repeat in the opposite direction.

Now articulate the feet slowly from flex through point and then back again. Repeat 10 times. Be aware of how the muscles in the feet work and contract to do this.

Home Feet Exercises

These exercises are for flexibility, strength, and comfort.

Ankle Circles - Sit in a straight-backed chair with your feet bare. Hold your feet slightly off the ground and slowly circle your ankles to the right and then to the left. Go as far in each direction as you can.

Towel Grabber - Sit in a straight-backed chair with your feet bare. Spread a towel out in front of your chair. Place your feet on the towel with your heels on the edge closest to you. Keep your heels down. Scoot the towel back underneath your feet by pulling it with your toes as you arch your feet. When you have done as much as you can, reverse the toe motion and scoot the towel out again.

Marble Pickup - Do this exercise one foot at a time. Sit in a straight-backed chair with your feet bare. Place several marbles on the floor between your feet. Keep your heel down and pivot your toes toward the marbles. Pick up a marble in your toes and pivot your foot to drop the marble as far as possible from where you picked it up. Repeat until all the marbles have been moved. Reverse the process and return all the marbles to the starting position. Note: If marbles are difficult, try other objects like jacks, dice, or wads of paper.

Foot Roll - This exercise stretches the ligaments in the arch of the foot. Sit in a straight-backed chair with your feet bare. Place a rolling pin (or a large dowel or closet rod) under the arch of your foot and roll it back and forth.

Meditation

The road to real health begins with the mind. Many people in western society start out with good intentions; perhaps the incentive is a heart attack, or something more basic like seeing themselves as they really are. Usually they go on a crash diet and embark on a heavy exercise program. If they don't kill themselves by the time they have lost weight they are too sick to enjoy it. Usually the 'fad' only lasts for a short while and the 'cravings' come back with a vengeance — so the patient is sicker than before because of the shock the system has sustained.

The only tool we have to make us stick to our intentions is the mind. Unfortunately the mind is usually in the same condition as the rest of the system through bad eating habits, bad thinking habits (aggravated by bad eating habits) and bad exercise habits. We need something to heal the mind first so that the mind can heal the body.

The area test influence on the mind is the way we live. Tension created by just living in the twenty first century is the greatest cause of ill health, and not many people realize this. We may be given a pill to ease the tension, but this does nothing to attack the cause of the tension and so the disease grows.

Around our bodies we have channels called meridians through which energy flows, something like the vessels through which the blood flows. All eastern philosophies of health talk of such a flow The Indians talk of Prana, the Japanese call it Ki, the Chinese call it Ch'i, and we call it electricity or life-force. The fact that it exists is not the question for most western people, but what is not known is how to keep a plentiful supply and how to keep the channels open.

What is needed is some way to train the mind not to allow tension to affect us. Whether the tension is psychological or physical it has the same effect on the body's energy. If the body's energy flow is interrupted or slowed down our natural healing systems are unable to cope with normal external attacks. Tension, more than anything else, affects the flow of Ch'i by closing the channels. Through the miracle of television cameras we can actually see the stomach contracting and unable to digest when the person is placed under stress or even thinks about being angry. The same things happen to the acupuncture meridians; they contract, allowing only a small amount of ch'i to flow to all parts of body. This can be used to great advantage by a trained martial artist; it is possible to strike certain parts of the body when the most ch'i is flowing through that area, to cause immediate great tension, thus closing the meridian. After some time, perhaps days, the meridian slowly closes completely and the recipient of the blow dies. This is sometimes called the delayed death touch or 'dim-mak'. However, it is said that this practice takes around three lifetimes to learn so not many ever come to such a level.

There is a small gland at the base of the neck running to the sternum. It is called the thymus gland, and in Chinese medicine is said to control the flow of ch'i as well as its physical function of producing anti-bodies. The first gland to be affected by stress is the thymus. The energy system of the body is affected immediately and if left unchecked will lead to the destruction of the body's energy system.

We do gain some relief from stress through sleep, but most of us counteract the benefit by sleeping on soft mattresses and watching television and eating before retiring. We need sleep to recharge our batteries; if we are using energy for digestion or for processing thoughts, we aren't using it to recharge. If we can find a way to stop stress from affecting us we are on the way to defeating the main cause of disease. We need to develop a calm mind, not always an easy thing to do. Meditation is completely foreign to most westerners, but Chinese exercises do not seem so strange because we are using the body to gain a mind effect.

Levels of meditation

There are three levels of meditation we can practice using movement. There is another, which requires no movement and is common to most forms of Indian yoga. This is where we sit cross-legged and meditate on a mantra or an object. Most westerners find this quite difficult, and can sometimes fool themselves into thinking that they are meditating. Moving meditation, although involving learning certain patterns of movement, can be easier because it does not use mind games. All we have to do is to learn and practice the movements in the correct way and the meditation will happen by itself; the mind will relax, the body will relax and as the body relaxes so too does the mind, and so on.

The first level of moving or 'working' meditation is where we stand in a certain position with slightly bent knees. This is the 'work' part of the meditation. The bent knees provide the heat necessary for certain chemical or energy changes to take place. It is not too difficult to maintain this sort of meditation but it is a little more physically difficult than the sitting kind. We are trying to teach the mind to relax while working. In this way we do not need a nice quiet room with candles in order to relax — we are teaching the mind to relax at all times so that tension does not build up. The basic stance for this kind of meditation (ch'i kung or Qigong). The legs are slightly bent with the knees not projecting any further than the toes. The toes are turned under a little, but not enough to make them turn white. The arms are held at chest height with the fingers pointing to each other. The fingers are held slightly apart with the palms concave. The tongue is pressed lightly onto the hard palate with the chin pulled in slightly to straighten the back. The eyes are looking straight ahead but not staring. The shoulders are relaxed with the elbows hanging. The breath is deep but natural and not forced, breathing in through the nose and out through the nose. This posture is held for at least 15 minutes but beginners can start with 5 minutes. Older people can practice this meditation sitting in a chair.

The second type of meditation is where we start to move while still holding the same relaxed meditative state induced by the Qigong. The slow, natural movements of T'ai Chi lend themselves to meditation, as there are not fast or jerking movements. The whole set is made up of different postures linked together by circling movements. One is able to keep a relaxed calm mind while performing the T'ai Chi form which lasts up to one hour. The movements relax the mind, this causes our movements to become more relaxed and smooth which in turn helps the mind to relax even more, so the mind and body help each other up the ladder

The third area of meditation is where we learn to perform more normal tasks while still holding the meditation. T'ai chi has another form of exercise called pauchui form, or cannon fist form, and as the name suggests this has some fast and hard movements. This form teaches us to keep our meditation even when confronted with the worst tension out in the street. In practicing this form while relaxed we are able to walk out into the big world knowing that nothing will upset us or make us tense.

Qigong

Qigong, or ch'i kung, translated means breath work or breathing exercises and we can use it to build up our internal energy or ch'i. We need an adequate supply of ch'i to each organ to maintain good health, but just as important is the free flow of this energy through the meridians.

In China there are Qigong clinics where people can go to be treated with Qigong either by a doctor or as a self help exercise. The patient learns the Qigong exercises so that self-healing takes place and this is obviously the best way. If however the patient is in no fit state to perform the exercises, then he must first be treated externally. This involves the doctor 'putting in' his own ch'i into the affected part or into the whole body.

If we are to heal ourselves we need a normal flow of ch'i, but if we are to heal others we need an extra amount of ch'i. This means that we ourselves must be fit and healthy, and apart from building up an extra supply of ch'i, we must also learn how to put it into others. This is a very simple practice physically but is quite difficult to learn mentally.

In order to heal others with ch'i we must know the meaning of yin and yang and how to cause different parts of the body to become yin or yang by using the mind. Once this is known, usually after many years of practising an internal art such as T'ai chi ch'uan or Taoist yoga, we then have to build up our supply of ch'i and learn how to get it into another person. A Chinese doctor confronted with a mild disease will stand in a Qigong posture for around 10 minutes to build up his immediate supply of ch'i. When he knows that he has enough to give he will either place one palm onto the affected area, use point massage, acupuncture or tui na (Chinese massage). All of these healing arts make use of 'putting the ch'i in'. The first method uses a point called pericardium 8, near the centre of the palm.

This is the healing point and is where the ch'i is able to escape and enter another either for the purpose of healing or in the martial arts. Point massage uses acupuncture points, pressing the relevant ones with the fingers and 'putting the ch'i in'. Acupuncture also uses this putting in of ch'i via very fine needles. The acupuncture point is activated by the needle and then the doctor puts the ch'i in via the conductor. This is a more effective way of getting the ch'i in as the electrical resistance of the skin is overcome. Tui na is a massaging technique that makes use of points and squeezing, manipulating techniques.

If someone has to be treated for a major ailment the doctor will fast or only eat fruit for 10 days and practice Qigong three times each day for at least 20 minutes each time. Only in this way will the doctor's body and mind be strong and clean enough to perform the difficult healing session. A great amount of energy is also needed for this session, hence the long Qigong.

Sometimes western students of Chinese healing methods only look at the physical effect of the particular practice i.e. they only study the technique of needling or the technique of massage. But if no ch'i is present then all of that learning is wasted. Some form of internal art must also be practised in order to gain the idea of ch'i. Qigong is the starting point for this learning.

History and origin of Qigong

The qi part (or ch'i) of Qigong means air or inner vital energy. Translated into western medical terms it means resistance to disease, adaptability to the external environment and the ability to overcome internal troubles and regain health. In Chinese medicine for thousands of years great importance has been placed upon exercises that strengthen the vital energy.

Traditionally any exercise that dealt with breathing and internal methods was considered to be Qigong. Nowadays we tend to call the more static breathing techniques Qigong and the moving exercises by their specific names.

The content of Qigong is varied but it mainly involves the regulation of the structure (posture), regulation of the mind, regulation of the respiration, self-massage and movement of the body.

The earliest records of Qigong come from the jin wen (writings on bronzes) from the Zhou dynasty (ca. 1100 —221 BC). During the Warring States period (770 — 221 BC) Qigong developed as never before and many great thinkers emerged. In the Book of Changes or I jing, semen, internal energy and the mind were considered to be the treasures of the body. An exercise akin to Qigong called daoyin was popular at this time. An inscription on a relic found in the Warring States period read, 'Take a deep breath and sink it to tantien (a point about 3' below the navel). Hold it there for a while and then exhale it as sprouting grass until it reaches the top of your head. This causes the Yang energy to rise and the Yin energy to drop. Those whose Yang and Yin energy goes its own way will live, otherwise you will die'. This saying was part of the daoyin exercise and holds true for all Qigong nowadays including T'ai chi, pa-kua, Taoist yoga and all of the internal arts.

In China today Qigong clinics have been set up to study and teach Qigong and to treat disease. Modern instruments have been used to detect infrared electromagnetic waves, and magnetic information coming from the palms of Qigong masters who are using this internal energy to treat such diseases as high blood pressure, neurosis, functional disease, paralysis, cerebral concussion and tumors of the thyroid gland. It is sometimes used as an anesthetic, although I'd want to be very sure it worked before it was used on me!

Healing yourself with Qigong

Qigong can be performed anywhere at any time and only takes around 15 minutes per session. At first you will need a quiet place where you are able to concentrate, but after some time you will be able to perform it in any environment, even on a bus or train if you don't mind people staring at you.

The postures

Three basic Qigong postures can be held — standing, sitting or lying down. The standing posture was described in Levels of meditation, see photograph 1. The sitting posture is much the same — sit on a chair with feet flat on the floor and the back straight. One of those old wooden kitchen chairs is ideal. Hold the palms in front as for the standing posture and vary the intensity by either moving the palms out for more effect or pulling them in if the exercise becomes too tiring. Clear the mind and concentrate on getting the breath down.

The lying position requires the same mind attitude as the others, but is good for the elderly and those in poor health. Lie on your bed or on the floor. Hold your palms over your chest with fingers pointing towards each other. You may vary the intensity by lifting your arms higher, or holding the palms further apart. A subconscious flow of ch'i should be felt in the palms i.e. as if the palms want to move themselves in and out with the breath.

Four different palm positions

The palms can be held in four positions. The main position is called 'The Mother Position' and is the one seen in the photographs, with palms towards you. This position is a general health giver for the whole body and mind.

The second is its opposite, 'The Father Position' where the palms face outwards — everything else is the same. This causes the ch'i to flow into different muscles. This position is used when 'Yin sickness' occurs i.e. where a person has not much energy, is too thin, out of condition from too much softness.

The third position is 'The Daughter Position' where the palms face downwards as in photograph 5. This position is used to cure any arm, wrist or palm injuries, including arthritic complaints.

The fourth position is 'The Son Position' and is seen in photograph 6. The palms are facing each other and bent slightly at the wrists, but not enough to cause tension. This position treats ailments of the upper back and arms.

Moving Qigong

Any movement that uses relaxed postures integrated with breathing techniques could technically be called Qigong. However there are certain exercises that also work on specific organs or in the treatment of certain diseases when combined with the breathing techniques.

The changing of the sinews, or triple warmer Qigong

This triple warmer exercise is said to balance the yin and yang energy of the body. Stand in a normal position with feet relaxed, toes turned slightly outward. Breathe in through the nose and lift both palms up in front of you with the palms facing upwards. The fingers point towards each other as you stand up onto your toes. Older people may prefer not to stand on their toes.

As you breathe out, turn the palms downwards still with the fingers of each palm pointing towards each other and push downwards back to the starting point as you lower your heels. This must be done with very relaxed palms and shoulders. Make sure the shoulders do not lift up at any time.

This first movement is called the Lower Warmer and acts upon the elimination organs, colon, kidneys, etc. Repeat this exercise three times and then go on to the next part, called the Middle Warmer. This exercise acts upon the digestive organs.

This time lift the palms in the same way as before, coming up onto the toes again. This is exactly the same as before. Now as you breathe out, turn both palms outwards at chest height and push out away from your body. When you push out from your chest, the arms should be held at arms length but not quite straightened. Continue the push until the palms have reached the sides of your body. Continue the circular movement and push downward at both sides until the palms have come back to your hip level. Remember to stay relaxed.

For the Upper Warmer, start the movement in the same way as for the other two by bringing the palms upwards and standing up on your toes. This time gently roll the palms up and over your head with the palms turned up. Hold your breath as you push upward. Next, take both palms out to either side and as you push down, breathe out and stand down. This acts on the respiratory system and the mind.

Never eat before or after practicing any Qigong for at least 10 minutes and preferably one hour as digestion uses up too much energy The main areas of energy use are procreation (sex), digestion and physical or mind movement. So when practicing any meditation we need the ch'i to flow freely. If we use up the gained energy there is no sense in doing the exercise in the first place.

Exercise for the alleviation of the triple warmer

This exercise harmonizes the three vital forces, respiration, digestion and reproduction. Link your fingers down near the tan-tien (3' below the navel). As you stand up in the same way as for the first triple warmer exercise, bring the palms up to chest height, this time a little closer to the chest. Photograph 14. Now push both palms up over your head as you look at the backs of the palms, which have been turned outwards. Hold this position for about 5 seconds and breathe out as the palms part and push down to either side. Harmonizing yin and yang of stomach and spleen

This exercise works upon the stomach and spleen, which are linked in Chinese medicine. Lift the palms as before with the fingers almost touching and the palms in close to the chest as you breathe in. Now push one palm up over your head, palm up, and one down to your side, palm down. Hold this position for about 5 seconds while holding the breath and then breathe out as the upper palm comes down to the same level as the other. Repeat this on both sides.

Prevention of tuberculosis

Turn your head as far as possible while breathing in. Don't strain. Hold this position for a count of 5 then turn back to the front while breathing out and repeat on the other side. Photograph 17 If any unusual amount of pain is felt in either shoulder as this is done, there could be something wrong with your small intestine.

To strengthen the kidneys

Bend down with knees straight, grab your big toes and lift them upwards as you breathe in. Hold this position for 5 seconds and breathe out as you stand up. Older people may bend the knees. This exercise acts upon the kidney meridian. See photograph 18. An alternative is to simply press the main kidney point called K1 on the sole of the foot just between the mounts of the big toe and second toe. Hold pressure for 7 seconds and stop, then repeat.

For daily meditation, try the following: Have someone read the following to you in a gentle, slow voice, clueing you as to the steps. You can also tape this in your own voice and listen to it as you go through the meditation. Eventually you will be able to go through the steps silently.

Sit comfortably in a chair or lie down on a mat on your back.

Allow your body to begin to relax. Close your eyes. Close your mouth and place the tip of your tongue against the roof of your mouth — this connects the Yin and Yang channels and allows for Qi flow.

With your eyes closed, bring your attention to the area around and below your navel; in Japanese it is called the hara; in Chinese the dan tien. This is one area where Qi is stored.

Allow yourself to begin to breathe into the area. You may use either breathing technique.

And as you breathe into the abdomen, into the belly, into the dan tien, notice a warmth from the center of the abdomen, beginning as a small glow and getting brighter and brighter until there is a ball of light filling your abdomen. Allow yourself to feel this ball of light, any color that you'd like.

Now, as you breathe, notice the energy moving up into the area of your heart and opening up into your chest.

Now feel it move to the area in front of the arm, just below the shoulder bone. This energy moves from the area below the shoulder bone, down the outside the arm all the way to the thumb, on the inside of the thumb.

Feel the warmth and the movement of energy down this channel.

When it gets to the end of the channel at the tip of the thumb, move your focus over to the index finger, where the Large Intestine Channel begins.

The Qi then moves through the hand, up the outside of the arm, coming up over the shoulder, up the side of the neck, and up to the outside of the nose.

Then move to the Stomach Channel, which begins below the eye. It flows down the neck, over the front of the body, through the chest, down outside the navel, around the pubic area, then down the outside of the leg, to a very important point, just below the knee, where the energy of the body becomes very strong. It then moves on down across the front of the foot and into the top of the toes, where it meets the Spleen Channel.

The Spleen Channel allows food energy to move through the body and impacts digestion.

Begin inside the big toe, coming up the arch of the foot, in front of the ankle bone, on the inside of the leg, all the way up by the knee, continuing inside the leg, and up the front of the body, curving around the ribs, and ending in the sides of the torso, also known as the costal area.

The Spleen Channel then connects internally with the heart.

The Heart Channel emerges from the heart into the center of the armpit, moving down the inside of the arm, all the way to the small finger, where it attaches to the Small Intestine Channel.

The Small Intestine Channel is a very good channel to help open up the brain.

This channel runs up the outside of the arm, coming all the way back up, across the scapula, up the back of the neck and around the ear, where it ends in front of the ear.

This connects to the Bladder Channel, the longest channel, at the inside of the eye.

From the eye, the channel comes up across the top of the head, down the back of the neck where it splits into two parallel lines which they extend down the whole back on either side of the spine, connecting the organs together.

The two rows of the Bladder Channel are side by side, then connect again at the back of the buttocks, coming down the back of the middle of the leg through the knee, all the way down the leg, around the ankle bones and into the little toe.

The Bladder Channel connects with the Kidney Channel on the very bottom of the foot. The Kidney Channel moves up from the foot, around the inside of the ankle, all the way up the inside of the leg, up around the navel. And this channel comes all the way up to the upper part of the chest, where there are some of the most important points in Chinese Medicine for meditation and connection with the Spirit.

Here the Kidney Channel connects with the Pericardium Channel which starts in front of the arm, moves down the very middle of the arm, into the palm of the hand, to the middle finger, where it then connects with the Triple Burner Channel, the channel that helps to regulate the temperature of our bodies. This begins on the fourth finger, comes up over the top of the hand, all the way up the arm and around the elbow, over the shoulder, coming up the neck and around the ear, where it connects with the Gallbladder Channel.

The Gallbladder Channel is the most crooked channel on the body. It zigzags across the top of the head, comes down the back of the neck, across the shoulder, down the side of the body, zigzagging again on the side of the body, and all the way down over the hip and the deepest point in the muscle of the body in the buttocks, then moving down the side of the leg, all the way down to the top of the toes, to the fourth toe.

You pick up the Liver Channel on the big toe. It comes across the top of the foot, and again towards the inside of the foot and around the ankle, up the middle of the inside of the leg by the knee, all the way up the inside of the leg. This channel circles the genital area, coming up into the ribcage near the liver, yet on both sides of the body. And then we return again to the lungs.

Once you have completed the cycle, sit or lie peacefully, allowing yourself time to make the transition back to your surrounding environment in a graceful manner.

Breathing Activities

Breathing

You can learn how to breathe deeply from the abdomen. "During the forms, the even movement and rhythm are predominant," Lee says. "You learn to match your breathing with the movement. [There's no need to] consciously breathe in and out; there's only a general guideline. If you want to do a lower stance or do a movement more slowly, your breathing pattern changes. But you intuitively know how to breathe."

Since tai chi is a martial art, when you move forward and exert energy, you generally breathe out, Lee says, and when you move backward, you breathe in. "Your arm comes up, you breathe in, and your chest expands; your arm goes down, and you breathe out," he says. Lee does not advise students to immediately match their breathing with movement, because the movements themselves are already challenging enough to learn. Beginners often complain that when they move one arm, they forget the other arm, and when they master the arms, they forget the legs or their balance, he says. "There's really a lot of training. Do it slowly so you can maintain that total control and awareness."

Once a tai chi student masters the movement, he can think about matching the breathing more closely. But in the beginning, Lee advises: "Just breathe; let the wisdom of your body tell you when to breathe. When you run, you don't tell yourself, "Now I'm running, so I must breathe faster". The body picks it up anyway. When the body needs to breathe in, just inhale. When it needs to breathe out, just exhale."

Later in a student's training, usually during the second year, breathing and movement start to work with chi (internal energy) and the mind, Lee says. "It all focuses together like a magnifying glass concentrating nice, warm sunlight into enough heat to burn paper. You can generate tremendous power."

Does tai chi breathing practice have any direct application to other parts of life? "Abdominal breathing is basically a relaxed breathing," Lee says. "The basic movement of tai chi is raising and lowering the arm; it's called breathing in and breathing out. When [students] get stressed during the day, they should do some deep breathing to settle down. Immediately they can regain their calmness. Even three minutes of breathing can renew the strength. Tai chi, even without the movements, can immediately be applied to daily life.

The five major schools of breathing are medical, Confucian, Buddhist, Taoist and Wushu or martial arts. Medical breathing techniques aim at strengthening one's overall health and are mainly preventive. The Confucian school of breathing deals with self-cultivation and temperament. Taoist breathing deals with one's moral character and longevity. The Buddhist breathing exercises are broken into two lines of thought and involve mainly the mind. The first Buddhist school is called 'Samadhi' and claims that everything in the world is illusionary. The other school is that of meditation which deals with the cultivation of the mind and the preservation of all forms of life on earth. The Wushu method of breathing is for physical training and good health. All of these schools have one thing in common, that of training of the mind and development of the qi, or ch'i. The breath is the most important part of the Chinese self-healing arts. There are certain ways to breathe while performing the various exercises described in this book.

The first and most important way to breathe is the natural way i.e. we try to get our breathing back to a more natural way, the way of the child. As we grow older and are affected by stress, the cause of 70% of all modern diseases, our breathing rises to the upper chest and we end up only using the top portion of our lungs. The lungs start just under the collarbone and end at the bottom of the rib cage. But the major part of the lungs is the part covered by the ribs on either side of the abdomen. This part, through tension and stress is sometimes not used, and so we are only receiving a small amount of oxygen. We try to compensate for this by breathing faster. One of the big faults in western posture is the 'pull the belly in and stick out the chest' syndrome supposed to look good on men and women. But in order to pull in the stomach and stick out the chest we have to tense certain muscles and this restricts our lung capacity.

The first thing to do is relax the upper chest and shoulders so that the breath is able to go deeper into the lungs and eventually fill up the whole lung again.

If you find it difficult to relax the chest while standing in a Qigong position, lie down and place your palms across your stomach. As you breathe in, feel the lower abdomen pushing outward and try to totally relax the chest. It may not look too cosmetic but it may just save your life. Feel your palms rise with each breath and lower with each exhalation. Try to not force the action, just breathe and it should happen naturally IF YOU ARE RELAXED. If you have access to a small child, see how it breathes and copy that. If you have been doing heavy exercise then the chest may rise a little more with the breath, but generally the chest should not stick right out.

Breathe with your nose; that's what it's for - there are certain times when we breathe through the mouth and I'll cover these later. Try breathing naturally while doing the triple warmer exercise covered earlier — this tends to open the lungs more. And remember there is a natural wait from inhaling to exhaling unless violent exercise has been undertaken.

Natural breath

For spiritual stimulation and physical comfort, try using the natural breathing technique just described. Now we try to use the imagination to cause certain energy circulations to take place. As you breathe out, imagine some physical object, say a ball-bearing or a marble, rolling from the crown, down the centre of your forehead, right down the front of your body to a position about 3" below the navel. This is the tan-tien or psychic centre. Only use this on the out breath.

Reverse breath

This breath is said to aid digestion and enable us to circulate the ch'i around the 'upper heavenly circuit'. The physical movements of this breath are different to the natural breath just practiced. As you breathe in, pull the lower abdomen in and as you breathe out, push the lower abdomen out. This is reverse breathing. The visualization for this breath is to imagine the marble being sucked up along your backbone from just under the anus (CV 1). The marble continues along the backbone and up to the crown, then down to just where the tongue is touching the highest part of your hard palate. As you breathe out, the marble travels down the tongue and then down the front of the body to the tan-tien. On the next in breath you suck the marble downward from tan-ten to CV 1 and then back up the backbone as before. This is called the upper heavenly circulation — the backbone route is the yang meridian and the front is the yin meridian.

Harmonizing Breath

This breath is said to harmonize the balance of yin and yang in the body and uses the reverse breath to circulate ch'i around the 'macro cosmic circulation'.

The inhalation is the same as for reverse breath, but this time as you breathe out take the marble right down both thighs and over the large toe to Kidney point 1, mentioned earlier. As you breathe in the ch'i comes up along the back of both legs, joins at the coccyx, then up the backbone, and continues as for reverse breath

Pre-natal or Fetal Breath

When a baby is in the womb it uses reverse breathing, using the part of the abdomen under the diaphragm. This is called pre-natal; everything above the diaphragm is called post-natal. In order to mix the inner and outer breath, we must breathe like an unborn fetus as well as a young child. To do this we must perform both reverse and natural breathing. As you breathe in, suck in the lower abdomen under the diaphragm. At the same time the part of the abdomen on the top of the diaphragm is pushed out. Now as you breathe out, the lower abdomen is pushed out while the upper is contracted. This causes a sort of wave effect and when the lungs are at full inhalation, the pre-natal and post-natal ch'i is allowed to mix at the border of the diaphragm. This is because the ch'i in the pre-natal part and in the post-natal part flow in opposite directions. If we breathe normally, using only natural breathing or only reverse breathing, then the two kinds of ch'i would not meet. As you breathe out, a little of the outer ch'i is added to the inner ch'i, and that is how we build up our store of ch'i by breathing.

Turtle Breath

Tortoise breath is exactly the same as pre-natal breath, but you must hold the breath in before exhaling for a count of 10. This allows more ch'i to mix.

It must be noted that it should take around 4 years to reach the level of tortoise breath, allowing some months on each of the preceding breaths.

Cleansing Breath

This is one of the times when we use the mouth to breathe. Breathe in through the nose and out through the mouth. This is said to cleanse the body of impurities and relax inner tension and lower fever. Sighing is a spontaneous manifestation of this sort of breathing.

Tonic Breath

This is the reverse of the previous breathing technique. This time breathe in through the mouth and out through the nose. This is said to act as a tonic and build up the body. This breath is said to give more energy and improve blood circulation.

Eye Movements

Firstly, a lot of eye problems in later life are due to a loss of tone in the eye muscles. These muscles become rigid, and this loss of elasticity reduces the ability of the lens of the eye to focus at different distances. It also causes the eyesight to become weaker. These exercises tone the eye muscles up and keep them elastic. If you already have eye problems when you begin these exercises, you will find your eyesight improving after a few months.

Secondly, any eye tension present will tend to produce a general feeling of tension, due to the eye's connection to the brain via the optic nerve. What happens is that eye tension produces an increase in the nerve impulses in the eye muscles. This increase in nerve impulses travels along the optic nerve and bombards the brain, causing a general feeling of tension and anxiety. The eye exercises will reduce tension in the eye muscles, as well as reduce general tension.

It is best to do these eye exercises while lying down after you've finished the asanas. This way you're resting after the asanas and doing the eye exercises at the same time, thus reducing the time taken to do your yoga routine.

When doing the eye exercises keep your eyes open and don't move your head.

Sitting (as in the exercises for the neck given above), open your eyes, then check on your posture. Is your spine erect? Hands on the knees? Body relaxed? Head straight? That is how you should always remain while doing eye exercises. The whole body must be motionless; nothing must move except the eyes.

Raise your eyes and find a small point that you can see clearly without straining, without frowning, without becoming tense and, of course, without moving your head. While doing this exercise look at this point each time you raise your eyes.

Next, lower your eyes to find a small point on the floor which you can see clearly when glancing down. Look at it each time you lower your eyes. Breathing should be normal. In other words, you don't have to do deep breathing.

Exercise 1 — Move your eyes upwards as far as you can, and then downwards as far as you can. Repeat four more times. Blink quickly a few times 1 to relax the eye muscles.

Exercise 2 — Now do the same using points to your right and to your left, at eye level. Keep your raised fingers or two pencils on each side as guides and adjust them so that you can see them clearly when moving the eyes to the right and to the left, but without straining.

Keeping the fingers at eye level, and moving only the eyes, look to the right at your chosen point, then to the left. Repeat four times. Blink several times, then close your eyes and rest.

Exercise 3 — Choose a point you can see from the right corner of your eyes when you raise them, and another that you can see from the left corner of your eyes when you lower them, half closing the lids. Remember to retain your original posture: spine erect, hands on knees, head straight and motionless.

Look at your chosen point in right corner up, then to the one in left corner down. Repeat four times. Blink several times. Close the eyes and rest.

Now do the same exercise in reverse. That is, first look to the left corner up, then to the right corner down. Repeat four times. Blink several times. Close the eyes and rest.

Exercise 4 — This exercise should not be done until three or four days after you have begun eye exercises given here.

Slowly roll your eyes first clockwise, then counter clockwise as follows: Lower your eyes and look at the floor, then slowly move the eyes to the left, higher and higher until you see the ceiling. Now continue circling to the right, lower and lower down, until you see the floor again. Do this slowly, making a full-vision circle. Blink, close your eyes and rest. Then repeat the same action counter clockwise.

Do this five times then blink the eyes for at least five seconds.

When rolling the eyes, make as large a circle as possible, so that you feel a little strain as you do the exercise. This stretches the eye muscles to the maximum extent, giving better results.

Exercise 5 — Next comes a changing-vision exercise. While doing it you alternately shift your vision from close to distant points several times.

Take a pencil, or use your finger, and hold it under the tip of your nose. Then start moving it away, without raising it, until you have fixed it at the closest possible distance where you can see it clearly without any blur. Then raise your eyes a little, look straight into the distance and there find a small point which you can also see very clearly.

Now look at the closer point-the pencil or your finger tip then shift to the farther point in the distance. Repeat several times, blink, close your eyes and squeeze them tight.

Exercise 6 — Close your eyes as tightly as you possibly can. Really squeeze the eyes, so the eye muscles contract. Hold this contraction for three seconds, and then let go quickly.

This exercise causes a deep relaxation of the eye muscles, and is especially beneficial after the slight strain caused by the eye exercises. Blink the eyes a few times.

Exercise 7 — This exercise is called 'palming' and is very relaxing to the eyes. It is also most important for preserving the eyesight. Palming also has a beneficial, relaxing effect on your nervous system. It's an ideal way to finish off the eye exercises.

Remain seated on the floor. Draw up your knees, keeping your feet on the floor and slightly apart. Now briskly rub your palms to charge them with electricity and place the cupped palms over your closed eyes. The fingers of the right hand should be crossed over the fingers of the left hand on the forehead. The elbows should rest on your raised knees and the neck should be kept straight. Don't bend your head. Do the deep breathing while palming your eyes.

If you are going to do the palming for longer than a few minutes, better sit down at a table, place some books or pillows in front of you to support your elbows so that you will be able to keep the neck straight, and palm the eyes in this position. If the palming is done for only a short period one can do deep breathing for half a minute or so at first, gradually increasing it every week.

Benefits: This exercise helps to do away with eye strain, and tension. Your vision will get better and clearer as the ophthalmic, or eye, nerves receive a richer supply of blood. Some people use this to improve their vision.

Massages for the Body

There are two ways of using Chinese methods of healing. Both build up our chi or cause the chi to flow with T'ai chi or we can manipulate our own points. In self-massage we manipulate our points and stimulate the chi we already have. The first, more common way is to simply manipulate the various acupuncture points to cause them to activate. The second is Qigong self-massage. It is stimulating, relaxing, and helps your organs to detoxify, not to mention getting the qi flowing through your meridians, because we will be stimulating acupuncture points along many of your major organ meridians. You do not need to know exactly where these meridians are or which organ systems they are associated with; just do this full massage and you'll be sure to hit them all.

Method 1 — There is a set routine starting from the head and moving down. Follow the procedures as mentioned:

Sit on the floor in a lotus or cross-legged position. The palms are held as shown in photograph 35; the eyes are slightly closed with the tongue pressed lightly to the hard palate. The shoulders are relaxed and the back straight and vertical to the ground.

After a short time of meditation rub the palms together for about 10 seconds to create some heat. Then place the index and middle fingers of each hand onto the forehead. Rub the fingers back and forth lightly all over the forehead for about 10 seconds, then take the palms back down to the knees in a circular movement and meditate again for about 10 seconds, breathing deeply but gently.

Next, rub the palms together again and place the same fingers over each eye and rub gently for 10 seconds, covering the whole closed eye and the eye socket. Take the palms back to the knees. Rub the palms together again and take the same fingers up to the ears and rub the whole ear for about 10 seconds, including behind the ear and just down onto the jaw. Take the palms back down again and meditate. Rub the palms together again, and this time take the fingers around to the back of the neck rubbing gently the whole of the neck back and front and up into the medulla (back of the brain). Take the palms back to the knees. Rub the palms and repeat the whole process on the mouth and chin including the cheekbones.

To massage the head we start by rubbing the palms together and then leaning forward as we press the fingers of each hand into the floor for about 3 seconds. See photograph 37. Now take the tips of the fingers of each palm and tap the whole skull so that you feel the pressure is almost painful but not quite. See photograph 38. Take the palms back to the knees.

For the teeth, we 'clack' the jaw 36 times. With hands on your knees, open your mouth and clack your teeth together lightly Even if you have false teeth you will still be activating the acupuncture points of the jaw. This is important for the normal functioning of the bowel.

Next we rub the palms together, and this time using a closed fist rub the whole of one arm with one fist. The pressure should be firm. Repeat this on the other arm.

Bring the palms back to the knees and rub them together again. This time the closed fist rubs the whole chest area using both fists together.

Take the palms back and rub them again. Now take the fists around to your lower back and rub the whole of the kidney area

Take the palms back to the knees and repeat the rubbing together. Now place your left palm onto your left knee. Using the right thumb and forefinger, rub with a heavy action the point just between the thumb and forefinger. Repeat this procedure on each of your fingers, rubbing the whole way down to the tip with a little force. Then complete by rubbing the back of the left hand with the right palm. Repeat this procedure using the opposite hand. The same procedure is carried out on the legs. Using the closed fist lightly punch the underside of the thigh and rub the top of the thigh. The same applies to the lower leg. Rub the toes and when completed take a hold of each foot and shake it gently. Also press using a little force all over the sole of each foot using the tips of the fingers.

To complete the self-massage, place each fist onto your chest and breathe in. As you gently throw both fists out, bend at the waist as far as you are able and breathe out. Hold this posture for about 10 seconds before sitting up and breathing in again.

Stand up and in a very relaxed way and swing each arm in turn until the fist strikes the shoulder. You should feel a slight shock wave. Repeat this 3 times on each shoulder.

Method 2 — In Qigong self-massage is one of the essential foundations for health and longevity. If one is doing much sitting meditation, it is essential to do stretching and self-massage to loosen tight muscles, lubricate joints, and increase circulation. A basic full self-massage routine is as follows:

Sit comfortably in an upright position with the spine straight, such as on the edge of a chair or bench, or cross-legged on a cushion. Taoist texts often say: "Loosen your hair and your clothing." Undo your belt and unsnap your pants to allow your lower abdomen complete freedom to expand and contract during deep breathing.

Rub your palms together until they are hot. It's OK if it reminds you of Mr. Miyagi in Karate Kid!

Place your hot palms over your eyes. Circle your eyes three times clockwise and then three times counterclockwise. Press in with your palms around your eyes--eyebrow, cheek bone, and the sides of your nose.

Circle your palms out, rubbing your forehead (from the center out), temples, and then pull your hands down the side of your face to rub your jaw with your fingers.

Use your fingers to press points around your eyes--the inner corner, outer corner, under the eyebrows, directly below the eye.

Use your index fingers to massage firmly down the sides of your nose. Press in on the points by your nostrils where your smile line starts. Trace down your smile line (smoothing the wrinkles out of it) to the corners of your mouth.

Slide your index finger behind your ear while your other fingers are on your cheeks and temples. Massage your ear up and down like this a few times. Using your index finger inside your ear, trace around the contours. Insert your index finger into your ear canal a little ways, and pop it out.

Run your fingers back through your hair, combing your scalp and down the back of your neck a few times. Then rub your palms down the back of your neck to your shoulders 3 times.

Tilt your head back and rub with your fingertips down the sides of the front of your throat. Tap very lightly on your windpipe to activate the thyroid and parathyroid glands which are in your throat.

Cup your right hand and slap/tap your left shoulder, outer arm, forearm, and the back of your left hand. Go down and then back up. Try to reach over as far as possible to get the left trapezius and the top of the left shoulder blade (scapula). Turn your left palm up and then pat down the inside of your left arm. Grab your left hand with your right (left palm up, right thumb on top of the left palm) and massage the left palm with your thumb. Starting with the left pinky, massage and rub each finger, giving it a gentle pull or popping it. Turn the left palm back down and rub the tender point in the muscle between the thumb and first finger (LI-4, He Gu).

Repeat the arm/shoulder/hand massage on the right side using the left hand.

Use both palms to brush down the chest, breasts, and ribcage to the belly. Massage the breasts in circles a few times each direction. Use your palms or fingers made into a beak to tap along the borders of your lungs--under the clavicles, down the sternum (activating the thymus gland), and along the lower ribs (vibrating your liver, pancreas, spleen, etc.)

Raise your left arm and use your cupped right hand to slap the side of your trunk, from under the armpit down to the "love handles." Repeat this on the other side.

Make your hands into loose fists and tap your kidneys and low back with both hands at the same time. Use the flat surface made by the thumb and forefinger in a loose ring. If you cup your hands correctly, you'll eventually hear a sort of hollow sound from the striking of your hands on your back. Go up your back as far as you can, and then back down to your sacrum and hips.

Overlap your fingers and use them to massage your abdomen in circles, clockwise and then counterclockwise (as if you have a clock facing out from your belly with your belly button as the center). Take a deep breath, pushing out your lower abdomen, and lightly tap it with your palms.

Depending on how you're sitting, get access to your left leg. Massage the thigh with both hands, then make loose fists and tap them on the inner thigh, top of the thigh, and the lateral thigh. Grab your thigh with both hands, fingers curved around to the back of your thigh, and press in along the center line of the back of the thigh, from the back of the knee (popliteal fossa) then as far up as you can go towards where the thigh meets the buttocks.

Repeat the thigh massage on the right side.

Gain access to your left calf and lower leg. If you're sitting in a chair, cross the left leg over the right thigh. If you're cross legged, put the left leg on top (half-lotus) or put your left foot on the ground with your knee up. Use your thumbs to massage the inside and back of the calf. On the inner lower leg where the tibia ends and the muscle begins, there is a line which is generally tender upon deep pressing with the thumb. It's the spleen meridian, and a good one to massage regularly to help keep the circulation going in the legs (to prevent varicose and spider veins, etc.). Make your left hand into a loose fist and pound down the muscles on the outer side of the lower leg.

Rotate your ankle in both directions with your hands. Massage each toe individually, popping them if you do that sort of thing. Press in with your thumbs on the sole of your foot, not being shy of any tender points. Pinch the Achilles' tendon on both sides of the ankle. Squeeze and tap on the top of the foot. Make a loose fist and pound the sole of your foot.

Repeat the lower leg and foot massage on the other side.

If there is an area of your body that is calling for more attention, spend a couple minutes massaging it. You can rub your hands together again to gather heat and place your hands over the diseased area/organ you're working on. Visualize healing light emanating from your hands into the area.

Finish by placing your hands, one over the other, over your belly button. Visualize your body's energy being compressed and stored into a pearl of light in your lower abdomen. This is charging your Qi battery, and is the traditional way to end any Qi Gong exercise or martial arts routine.

Body Soaks (Baths)

The essence of traditional Chinese healing is to see the body as a harmonious whole. To convey a holistic view of life, inspiration from nature is used. Hence, the concept of Yin and Yang, which essentially means the cloudy side of the mountain (cool) and the sunny side (warm). Existence, in ancient Chinese thought, is the interplay of five elemental forces represented by the earth, metal, water, wood and fire. Body soaks include Herbal and Tea Soaks, Face Soaks, Foot Soaks, Sun and Air Soaks, and Morning Cold Rub and Air Soaks that will not only stimulate your skin, increase blood circulation, and relieve tension, but also provide numerous other benefits for your body, mind and spirit for the whole family.

Herbal Soaks or Tea Soaks

The herbal bath or tea baths were not new in ancient China. According to the Chinese history, that the ancient Chinese started adding herbs into bath water to treatment of certain forms of disease can be dated as far back as Shang Dynasty (1700 to 1027 BC). However, the main purpose of the herbal baths was to maintain health. The herbal bath or tea baths were used by the queen or all those beautiful women around the emperor in ancient China. The purpose of herbal bath or tea bath was to relieve stress relief or maintain the skin to slow down the aging process. To date, there are very high percentages of the research reports in herbal or tea published by the Chinese. When did people start using herb bath? It is believed that people learned of the herb bath before they learned of how to write. In the west, the herb bath was used for aroma. The herb bath remedies were believed to be in the Chinese literature since 4500 years ago however the only reliable references can only be dated at around 300 BC. The 1st literature from the west that indicates herb bath can be dated at 1st century. In any cases, the physical evidences that exist today indicate that human might know of herb bath as early as 3000 BC. The herb bath does not seem to have any discrimination. It started as soon as human civilization started. May be ancient people indeed knew things that we don't.

The tea bath helps maintain and improve healthy skin, hair, stress relief and exhaustion. The tea bath also believed to help resist cold and flu. Tealeaves provide fragrances to the bath water. In addition, tea leaves are good for the skin. Tealeaves cleanse the skin and remove fatty substances. Those with skin problems are greatly relieved by the tea bath. A daily tea leaf bath prevents cartelization of the elbow and heels. Some of the herbal baths are used as a treatment for certain forms of disease. Some of the herbal baths are used to maintain skin and slow down the aging process. Herbal bathing is the one of the best remedy against stress, anxiety, insomnia. Both herbal bath and tea bath help combat fatigue and energy loss. Tea pillows and herbal pillows are believed to help sleep easier. The tea bath and herbal bath will help to reduce weight. The Chinese believe tea baths and herbal baths will increase circulation that burns your calorie and results in loosing weight.

The following are just a few of the common herbs for herb baths:

Radix Ginseng — Radix Ginseng is a herbal medicine that commonly used for herbal bath. Radix Ginseng is one of the best herbal bath elements in helping stress relief. Radix Ginseng is usually used in combination with other herbs specifically designed for women.

Rose — Rose is a common herbs found in herb bath. Rose is believed be an antidepressant, antiseptic, sedative, aphrodisiac, tonic, astringent, and antispasmodic. The rose oil has been found effective in cases of depression, insomnia, impotence, skin care, nervous tension, feminine complaints, grief, sadness, and low self-esteem.

Tea — Tea is one of the elements commonly found in herbal bath. Tea can be used as "by itself" for tea bath however; it is common to use tea in combination with other herbs to get the best out of a good and relaxing hot bath.

Astragali's Radix — Astragali Radix is believed to be an anti-hypertensive agent. It does really well in stress relief. It is also a vasodilator agent. It will help body circulation. It helps in preventing allergic reacts. It is also a diuretic agent.

Lycii Fructose — One of the most common Chinese herbal medicine. It also commonly used in cooking. It is really mild herbal medicine. It will help circulation. It is believed to have the same effect as ginseng radix in many ways.

Zizyphi Fructose — Zizphi Fructose is believed to do really well in stress relief. It is also believed to be an anti-allergic agent. Many people believe zizyphi fructose is a natural herb that will help women improve their sex drive. It is used intensively for that purpose. It is one of the herbs that have been used in herbal bath for thousand of years by the Chinese.

Angelicae Sinenesis Radix — Angelicae Sinenesis Radix is one of the most widely used herbs. It is useful to add in remedies for afflictions of the respiratory system, as well as liver problems and digestive difficulties. This herb promotes circulation and energy in the body. It is often used to stimulate the circulation in the pelvic region and to stimulate suppressed menstruation.

Artemisia Vulgaris — This is a herb used intensively for woman. It is believed to have abilities in healing many of the women's ailments and disorders. It is a natural antiseptic agent. It used intensively for women's remedies in Chinese medicine.

Jasmine— Jasmine is a common flower in Japan and China, The flower is usually mixed with tea for drink or for tea bath. Jasmine oil is commonly used in massage and acupuncture. Jasmine is an excellent medicine for aromatherapy to treat depression and nerve conditions..

Lavandar — Lavandar (Lavender) is one of the most common herbs used in herb bath. It is used for it anti-depression, anti-tension and stress relief. Lavender's name is derived from the Latin verb "to wash". It was used by Romans and Greeks for its' fresh smell. It's aroma has both uplifting as well as balance effect.

Water Lily Pads — They are also known as "lotus leaves" by the oriental. The water lily pads were widely used in ancient China. The water lily pads were used as a rice wrap (similar to today's lunch box), tea, spice and herbal medicine. The lily pads are believed to be able to cure headache, flue and a whole lot of other diseases. It is used in herb bath as a stress relief agent.

Face and Foot Soaks

Face and foot herbal soaks were once popular in China especially with the Qing royalty during imperial times. Soaks keep the limbs smooth and flexible, improve circulation, reduce aches and pains and prevent arthritis. Among the herbs used are cinnamon twigs and angelica roots, which can promote circulation, remove excess dampness and 'wind' in the body and have the abilities to penetrate to the limbs extremities and muscles of both the face and feet.

Face Soaks — Begin by washing your face with cold water when the weather is warm. After your morning exercises rub your face, ears, head and neck vigorously with both palms until they are warm. Wring out a towel in cold water that has been soaking in cinnamon twigs and use it to rub your face, ears, and neck. Then take a deep breath, dip your face into cold face and breathe out into the water (that has angelica roots soaking for a one hour). Repeat as many times as you feel is necessary and then rub your face, ears, and neck with a wrung out wet towel. This process will stimulate blood circulation, prevent colds and stimulates the skin. You can alternate with hot water baths every other day to further stimulate your skin and increase blood circulation.

Foot Soaks — Begin by putting 4 tablespoons of sea salt using 2 liters or half a gallon of warm water gradually decreasing the temperature of the water until it has dropped to 16C (62F). Then dip your feet into the water and rub them against each other. Soak your feet in the water for 3 minutes, and then take out your feet and dry your feet with a towel and rub your feet vigorously to warm them up. Next, drop the temperature of the water again until it drops to 4C (40F). Before putting your feet in the foot bath rub your feet until they are warm, then dip your feet into the water and rub them against each other. Soak your feet in the water for a 3 minutes, and then take out your feet and dry your feet with a towel an do the same foot exercise as mentioned above to warm up. You can alternate with hot water foot baths every other day to further stimulate your feet and increase blood circulation and relieve tension in your feet.

Sun and Air Baths

Sun and air baths are important for reviving the dead skin and for keeping it in normal condition. They should be taken every day. This can be done in combination with your regular exercise program, but may be taken at a separate time and place. Vitality or life force comes to us through the sun; and the direct action of sun, light and air on the skin is very beneficial.

Do not expose your body to the direct rays of the sun for too long a time at the start, as the sun's rays have a powerful, stimulating effect. You should begin with moderate exposure and gradually increase until you get the amount suited to your individual condition. If no special provision is made for outdoor air baths, take all exercises nude before an open window. The cold spray or sponge bath taken during exposure to the sun and air will increase skin action. Let the body dry in the air, rubbing it with the hands to increase its magnetism.

Before going to sleep, take a short air bath in front of the open window. This may be combined with breathing exercises and or self massage but care must be taken not to drive away sleep by over-strenuous exercise.

Morning Cold Rubs and Air Baths

After your morning or evening bath exercise nude before an open window, if the outside temperature permits. Soon the circulation and skin action will improve to such an extent that you can do this without worrying in midwinter as well as in summer time.

After the cold rub, while taking the air bath nude before an open window, go through the breathing exercises that are discussed in this book. If possible, exercise from fifteen to thirty minutes. Also pinch, pull, slap and massage the fleshy parts of the body vigorously, from the feet up. Rub the back with a flesh brush or with a rough towel.

Begin with the lighter exercises and from day to day take more difficult ones. The time to be spent in exercise must be determined by your occupation and other individual conditions. Do not exercise immediately before or after eating, or when very tired.

Education of Wushu Today

The Modern Viewpoint

In one study, published recently in Medicine & Science in Sports & Exercise, volunteers age 58 to 70 who practiced Wushu roughly five days a week showed a 15 to 20 percent improvement in aerobic capacity and knee strength after one year. In a second study, presented at a meeting of the American Heart Association, older volunteers with elevated blood pressure who did Wushu for 12 weeks lowered their systolic blood pressure (the upper number) by 7 mm Hg – nearly as much as those who did a moderately intense aerobic-exercise program of walking and low-impact aerobics.

In our modern world we travel very much in the fast lane maintaining lifestyles that are often extremely hectic, and resulting in many cases in poor eating habits, too little exercise and a great deal of mental stress. It has been said that more than 50% of illnesses treated by modern doctors can be attributed to psychosomatic disorders or, directly or indirectly, to mental stress.

It is well known that mental stress can cause physical illnesses such as cardio-vascular problems and high blood pressure. Stress has been proven to cause increased blood cholesterol levels and even some forms of cancer. Thus mental stress has a very clear and direct relationship to total body health, causing not only mental but also physical illness.

In practicing Wushu the principle requirement is for the mind to be completely cleared of extraneous thoughts so that it can concentrate completely on the execution of the required movements. When performing Wushu, remember the mind must be in a relaxed, yet clear and alert state so that it can be used to direct and coordinate the movement of all parts of the body. Using the exercises and meditation techniques in this book, improves the central nervous system and mental relaxation. When Wushu is practiced properly, the muscles are gently stretched out and fully relaxed and it would be impossible to do this in a tense state of mind.

Practicing Wushu is also a pleasurable experience, giving the practitioner a feeling of comfort and improving their mood. The idea was verified through the recording of electrical brain waves (EEG) of two groups of people. One group consisted of regular practitioners of Wushu while the other group, a control group, were not Wushu practitioners. In the experiment the Wushu group recorded a larger number of alpha waves than the control group. The production of alpha waves, the study reported, signifies a state of "mental clarity and concentration," and subjects were said to be "highly calm and alert" and to have "improved or restored memory."

Consistent with this is the importance of the well being and education of today's children. It has been documented that our young people have a shorter attention span. Wushu uses interesting and enjoyable methods to keep young students attention and teach them the skills they can use for life.

It promotes non-violent resolutions to conflict. It helps children to explore and understand conflict through role-play and other exercises. Students develop confidence, self-discipline, and self control as they learn how to act and react to the world around them. Young students learn to respect and taught to return the same respect to others.

Wushu praises, encouragement, and positive reinforcement to support the values parents teach at home. Children learn the value of setting goals and how to develop the perseverance and discipline to achieve them.

The benefits of Wushu training for the whole family are innumerable. Whether you are six or sixty, the physical benefits are widely publicized and accepted; increased cardiovascular fitness, reduced risk of many diseases, weight control, increased flexibility, enhanced functioning of the metabolic, endocrine and immune systems, and many others.

Many of the physical benefits of Wushu also have psychological effects. For example, by improving your health, Wushu increases your "sense" of well-being. Wushu students are likely to report reduced tension or stress. The physical nature of martial arts can lower the risk of depression and increase self-esteem! Wushu training is also an excellent avenue to release aggression in a controlled environment, giving students an increased feeling of power and self-control. Wushu requires the physical movement of the entire body which helps develop self-awareness and an understanding of one's own mind.

Finally, the purpose of writing this book is to introduce you to 'Wushu' as a series of Chinese traditional exercises and activities which will add to your family time together and help to keep the whole family active. Through a series of detailed traditional and up to date exercises and movements learning Wushu can strengthen not only an individual's sense of physical well being but also a family's relationship.

Young people who practice Wushu with their parents become closer as a family. It is important to find an activity that the whole family can practice together anywhere, and anytime. Wushu can be done inside or outside the house or even on a family holiday, in the hotel.

Remember these 11 words of encouragement when practicing Wushu:

Balance
Character
Confidence
Defense
Flexibility
Focus
Fitness
Power
Strength
Speed
Spirit

Wushu can be fun for the everyone. Whether it's for competition, passion, exercise or bonding, Wushu today helps promote a sense of overall well-being and genuine fitness for you and the whole family.